Delicious EUROPEAN Summer

ANTONINA DURIDANOVA

Delicious European Summer

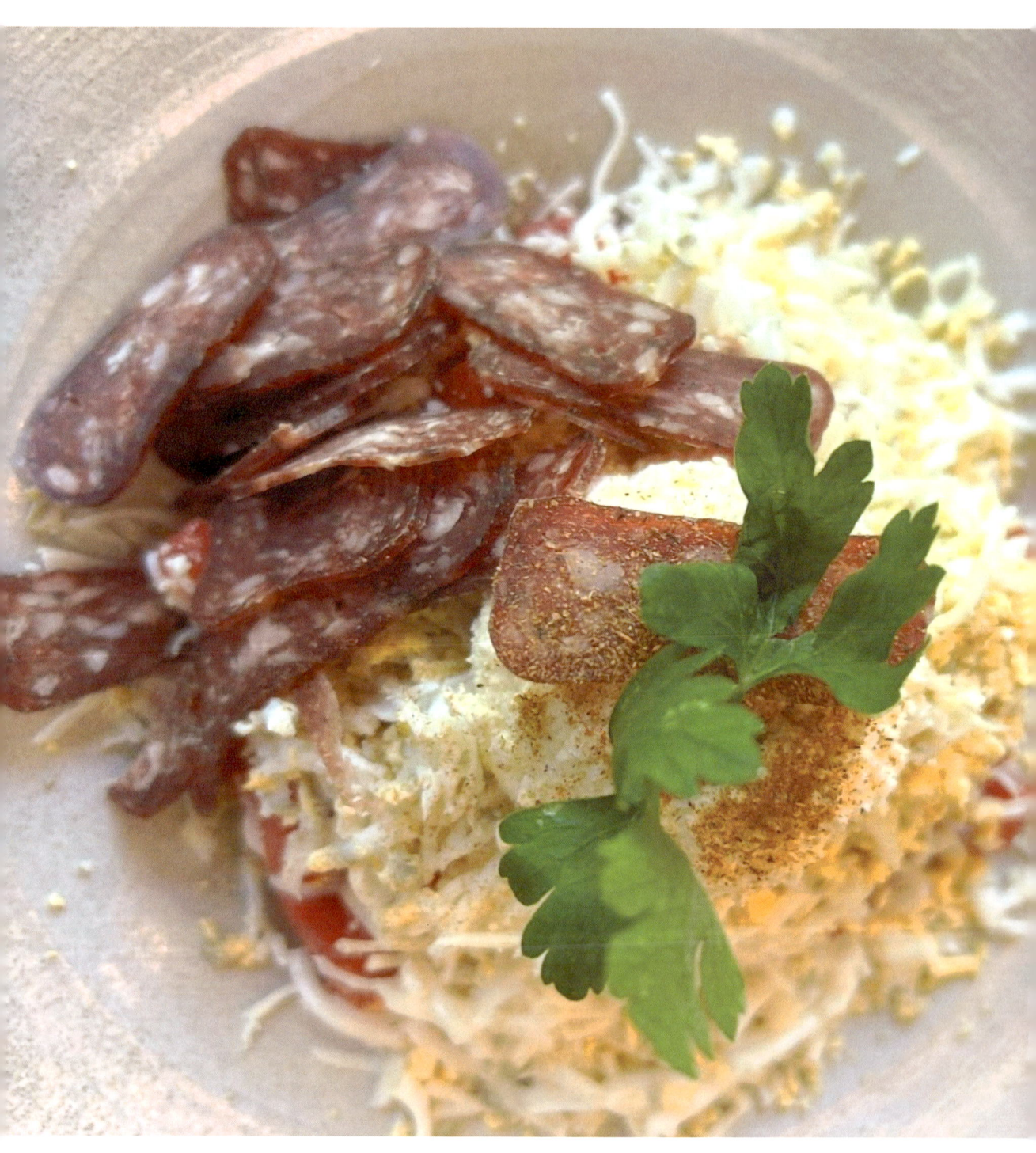

Appetizer

INGREDIENTS —————————————————————

1. Lukanka or dried salami, thinly sliced
2. One tomato, thinly sliced
3. Feta cheese – shredded
4. Kaskaval or yellow cheese – shredded
5. Slice of bacon – browned
6. Parsley

Arrange the serving plate by layering the sliced tomatoes on the bottom, sprinkle the grated feta cheese and yellow cheeses on top of the tomato slices, top with a slice of bacon, garnish with parsley and place the finely sliced lukanka or dry salami on the side.

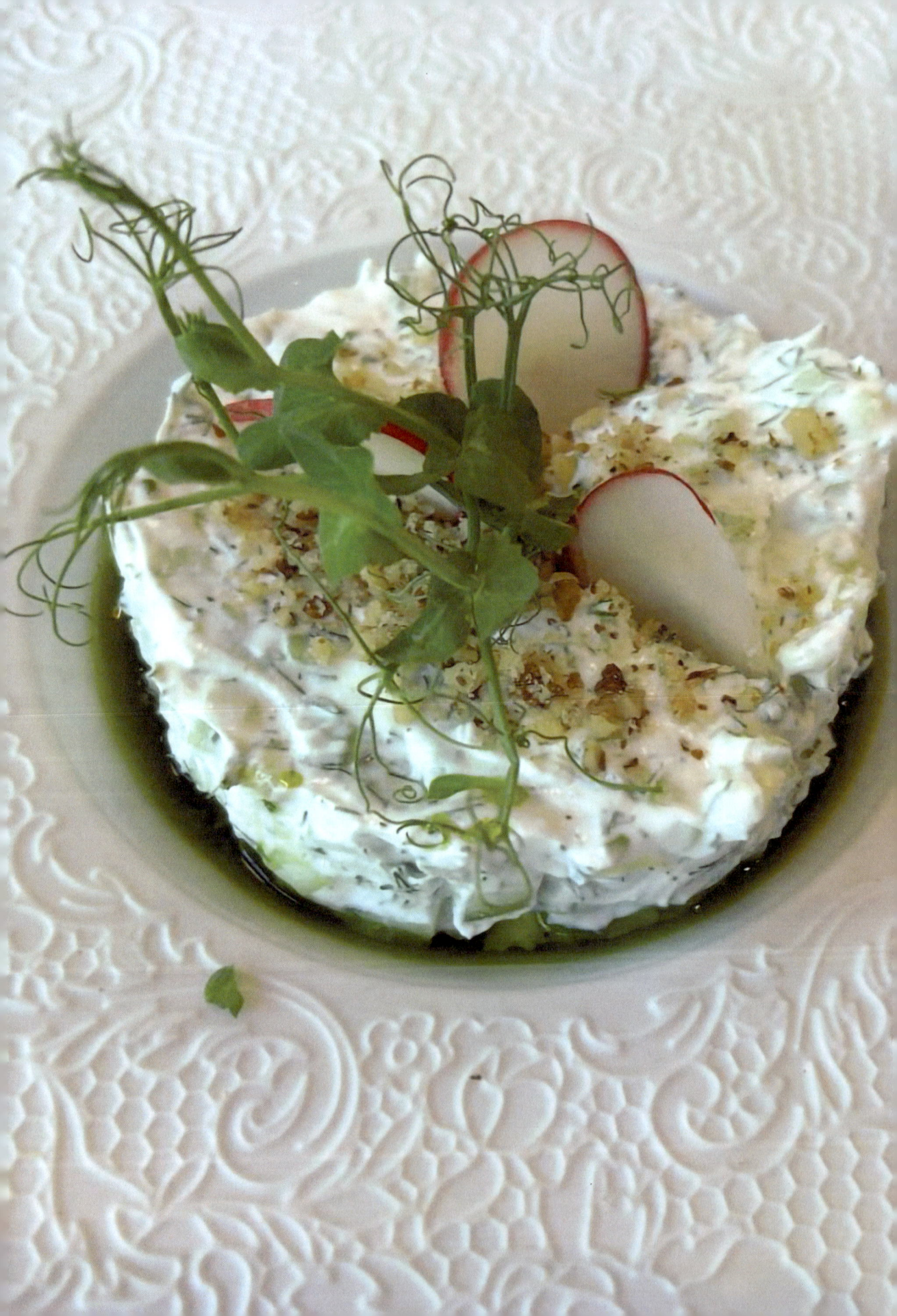

Appetizer Snezanka

INGREDIENTS ───────────────────────────────

1. Pickles
2. A jar of Greek yogurt, drained
3. Finely chopped/crushed walnuts
4. Radish for decoration
5. 3-4 cloves of garlic, crushed
6. Dill
7. Half a spoon olive oil
8. Arugula leaves for garnish

Mix the finely chopped pickles in the drained yogurt together with half the finely chopped walnuts, garlic, and dill, decorate with walnuts, sliced radish and leaves of arugula.

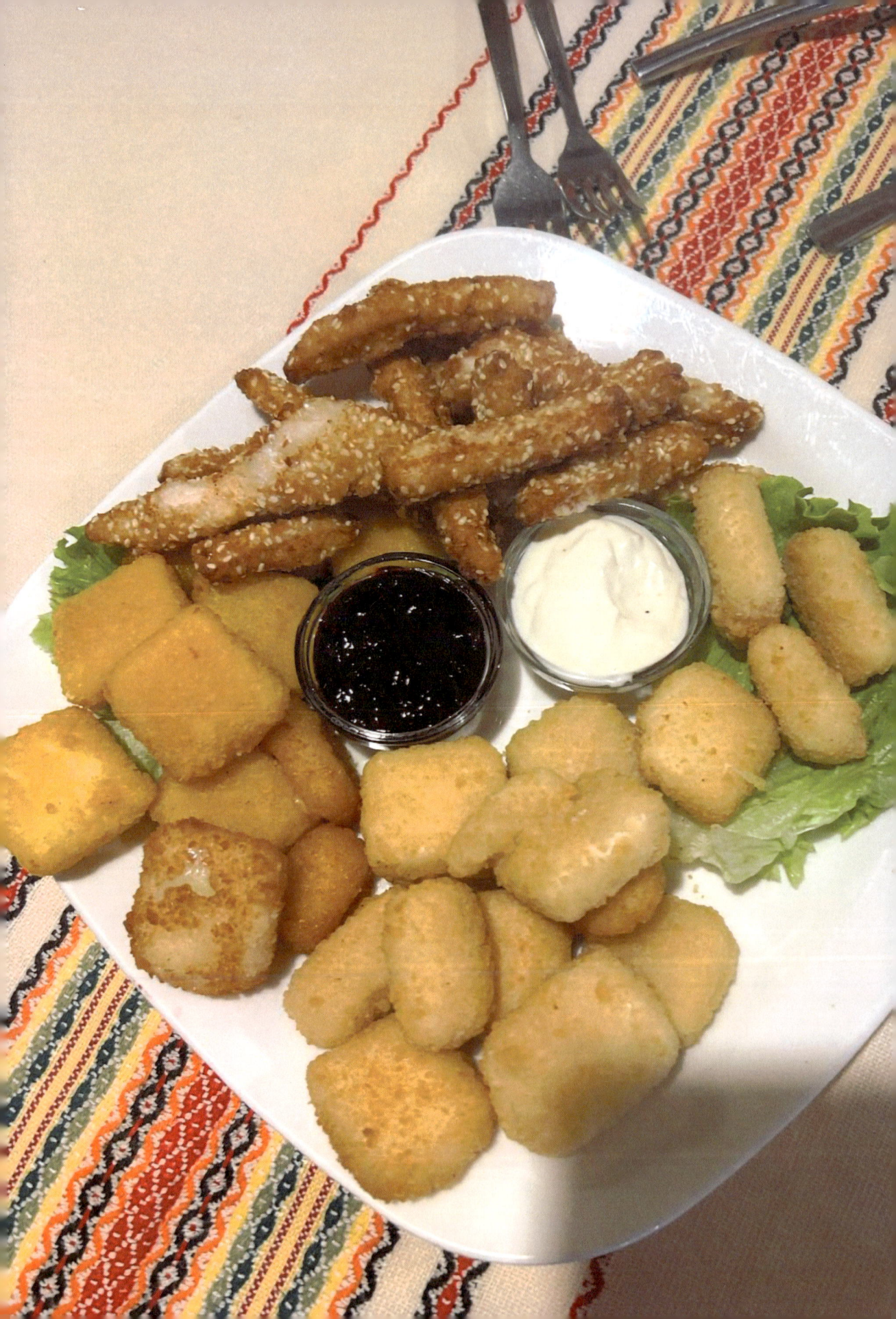

Kashkaval Bites And Solenki

Solenki

INGREDIENTS

1. Melted butter – 200 grams
2. Feta cheese – 100 grams
3. Milk – 100 ml
4. 2 eggs
5. Flour – 500 grams
6. Seeds – sesame or others
7. Baking powder – 1 teaspoon

In a bowl beat the eggs, add milk, the baking powder, part of the seeds, the grated cheese, and the melted butter (not hot). Add the flour and work it gradually into the mixture. Place the dough on a surface previously sprinkled with flour. Roll out the dough and make long or other forms that you like. Place the forms in a baking pan covered with baking paper, smear the mixed yolk of the eggs on the forms (solenki) and sprinkle with some of the seeds. Bake in a preheated oven at 360 degrees until golden in color.

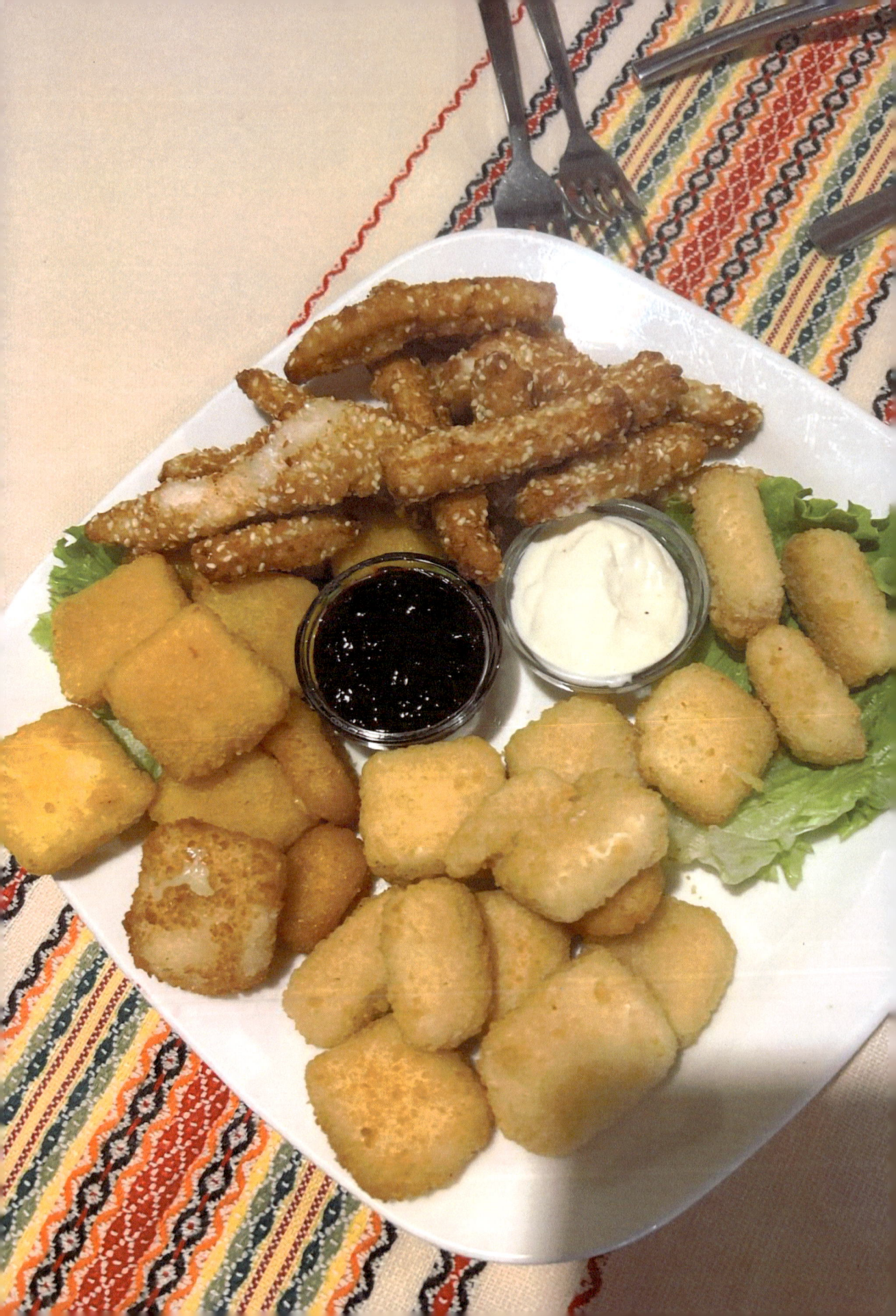

Kashkaval Bites

1. One-pound grated kashkaval (Bulgarian yellow cheese) or aged provolone, Italian caciocavallo or Greek kasseri.
2. Eight soup spoons flour
3. Two eggs
4. Teaspoon of baking powder
5. Olive oil

Add the eggs, the flour and baking powder to the grated cheese, and work into a dough; refrigerate for 20 min. Wet your hands and roll pieces of the dough into desired size kashkaval bites. Fry in a pan (for French fries) with heated oil until golden. Place the bites on kitchen paper to drain the oil.

Place the kashkaval bites and solenki on a dish and serve with dips of your choice.

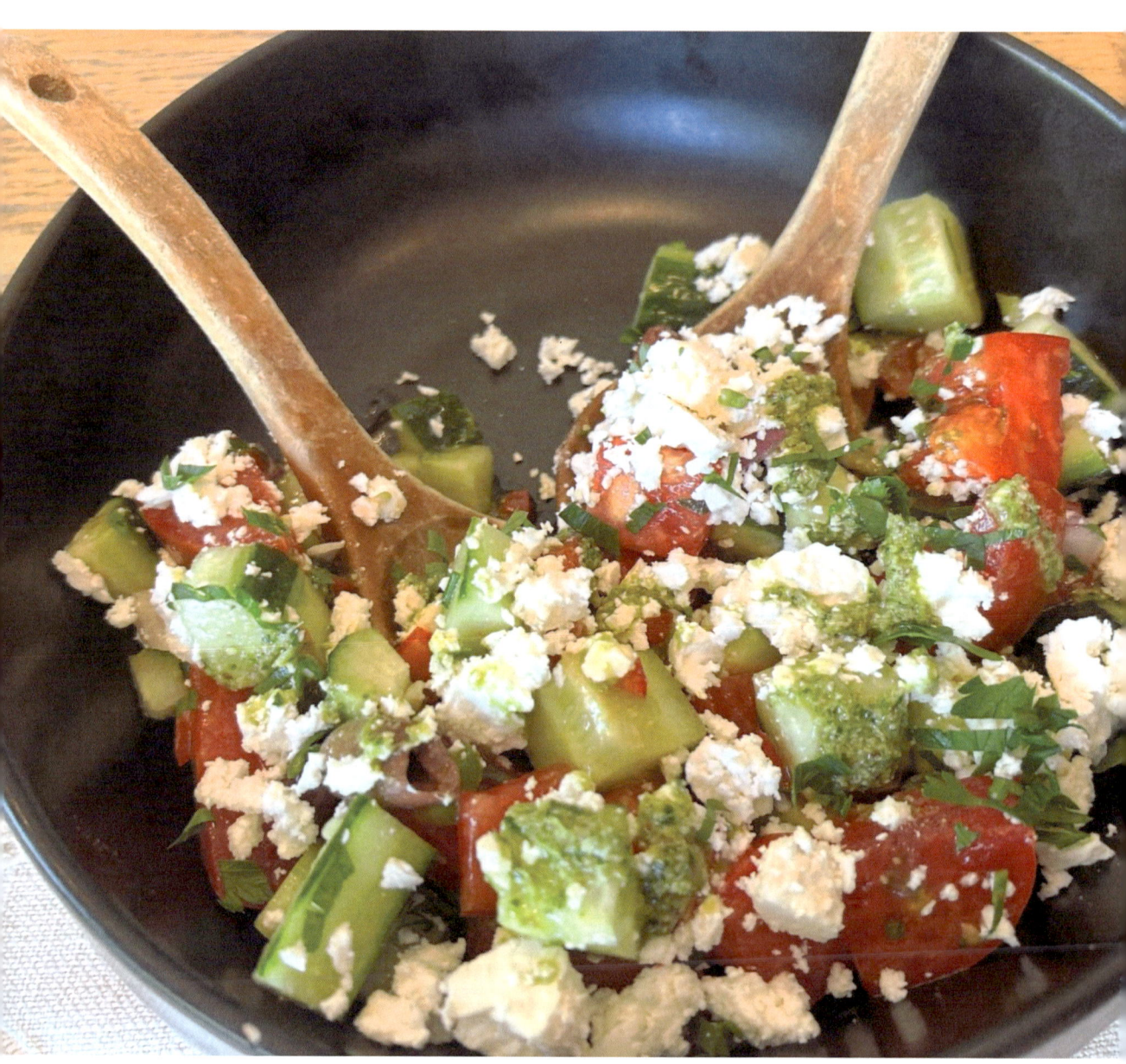

Summer Salad

INGREDIENTS

Tomatoes, cucumbers, spring onion, parsley, crumbled feta cheese, olive oil, squeezed lemon or lemon juice

Cut the tomatoes, cucumber, and fresh onion, and mix in a salad bowl. In another bowl mix a teaspoon of olive oil and juice of half a lemon, pour on salad and mix. Sprinkle on top the feta cheese and the cut parsley. Bon Appetit.

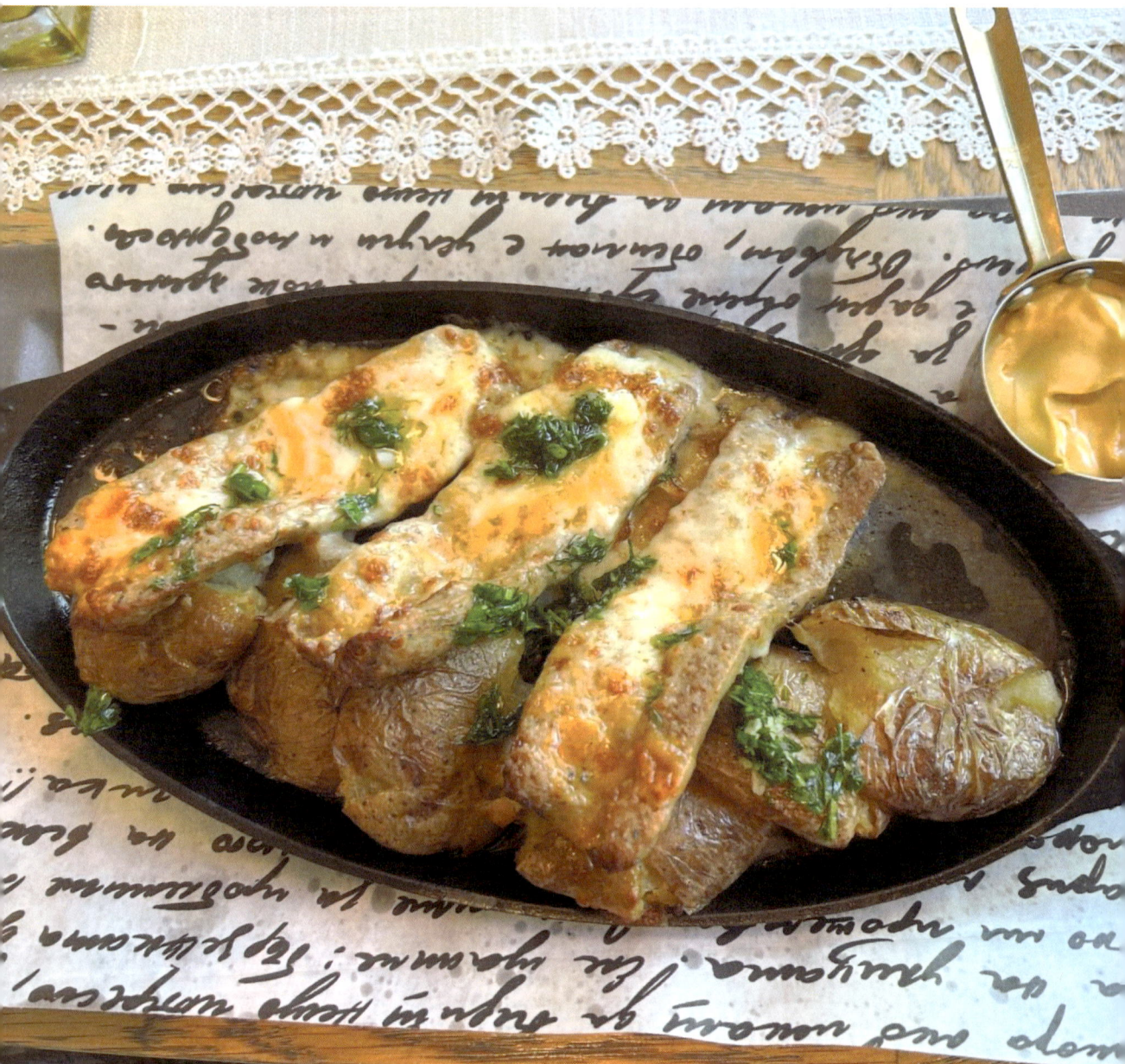

Specialty Dinner Dish Ingredients

1. Ribs – meat of your choice, marinated in olive oil, crushed garlic, lemon juice, salt and pepper, ½ teaspoon of cumin coriander powder and sweet paprika, add chubritsa or Italian seasoning.
2. Fresh small potatoes washed, not peeled.
3. Grated kashkaval or parmesan cheese.
4. Cut parsley
5. Dijon mustard, ketchup, and mayo.

Cut the upper part of the marinated rib and stuff with fresh potatoes. Wrap in aluminum foil and bake in a pan at 395 degrees for half an hour. Unwrap and sprinkle the grated cheese on top. Bake until cheese has a golden color.

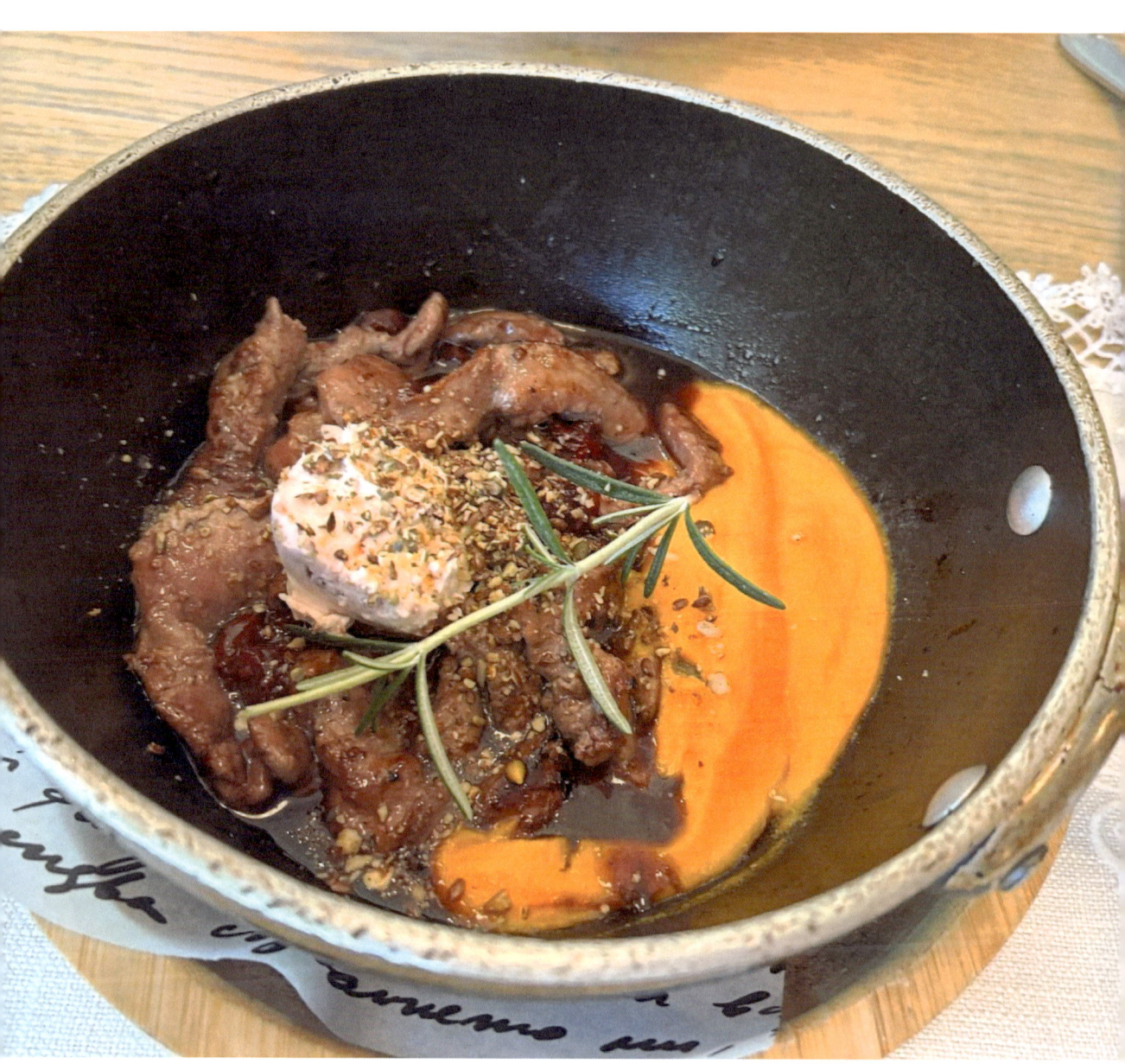

Kachamak/Polenta With Pork Bites

INGREDIENTS

Cornmeal, water, melted butter, salt, pork meat seasoned with salt, cumin, turmeric, sweet paprika, black pepper, feta cheese, powdery nuts of your choice, a piece of rosemary

I prepare polenta or kachamak in my rice maker, it's easy and it works. Add to the rice maker one cup of cornmeal, two cups of water, half a stick of melted butter, a pinch of salt, stir and let cook for 10 min. Stir constantly and make sure there are no lumps. When consistency is not watery, transfer to a baking dish for 5 min. to take the form of the dish. In the meantime, in a dish combine salt, black pepper, turmeric, cumin, sweet paprika. Cut the pork into strips and rub with the spices, roll the pork bites in flour and fry in a pan on the stove until it has color (do not overcook). Transfer the pork over the polenta, add a cube of feta cheese on top of the meat and bake on low – 290 degrees for 5 minutes. Take out of the oven and serve with a slice of feta cheese and a piece of fresh rosemary.

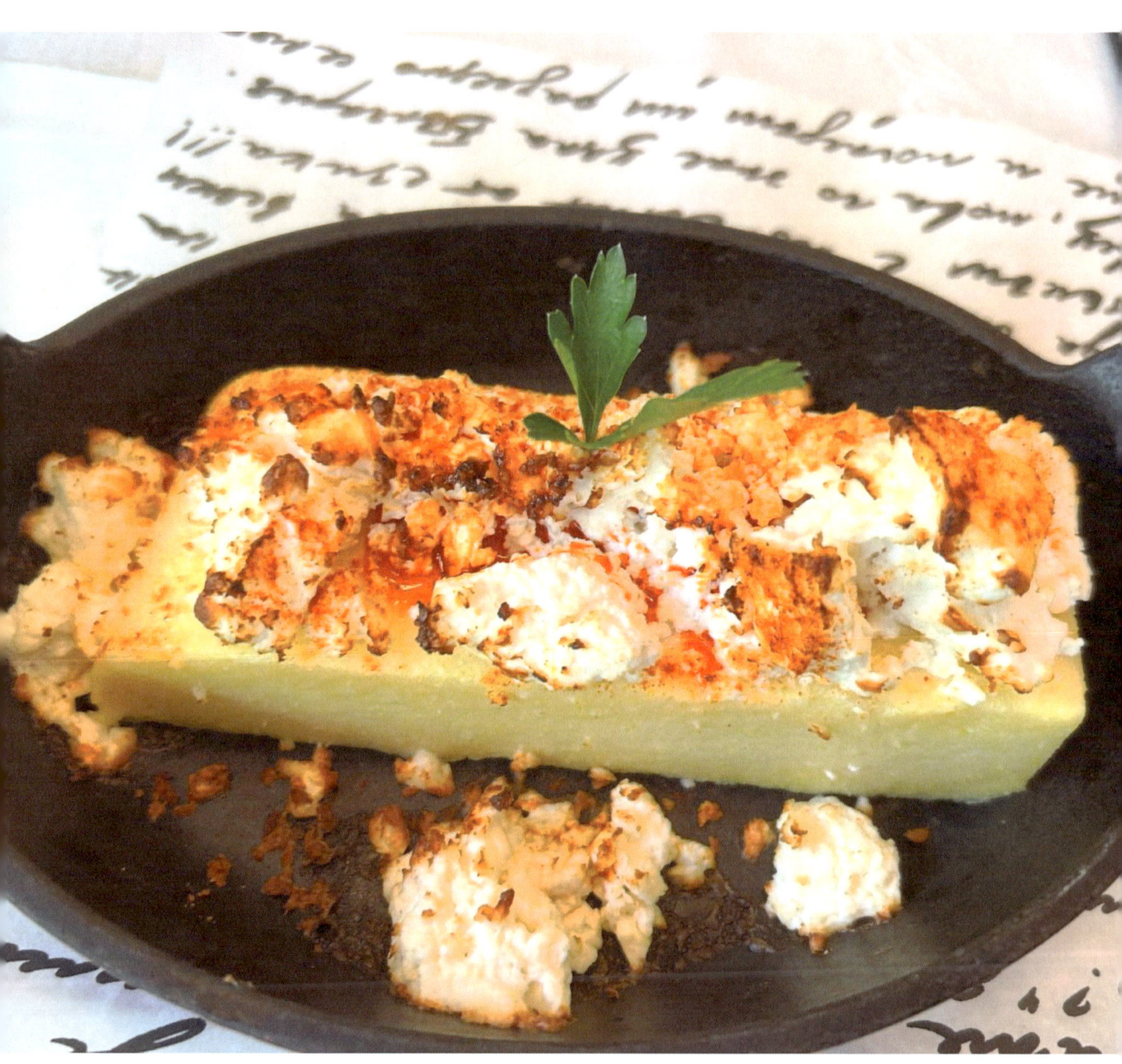

Kachamak / Polenta

INGREDIENTS

Same procedure as that for polenta with pork bites. On top of the polenta is chopped bacon or ham of your choice and more feta cheese, loosely crumbled and baked for a couple of minutes to slightly melt the cheese

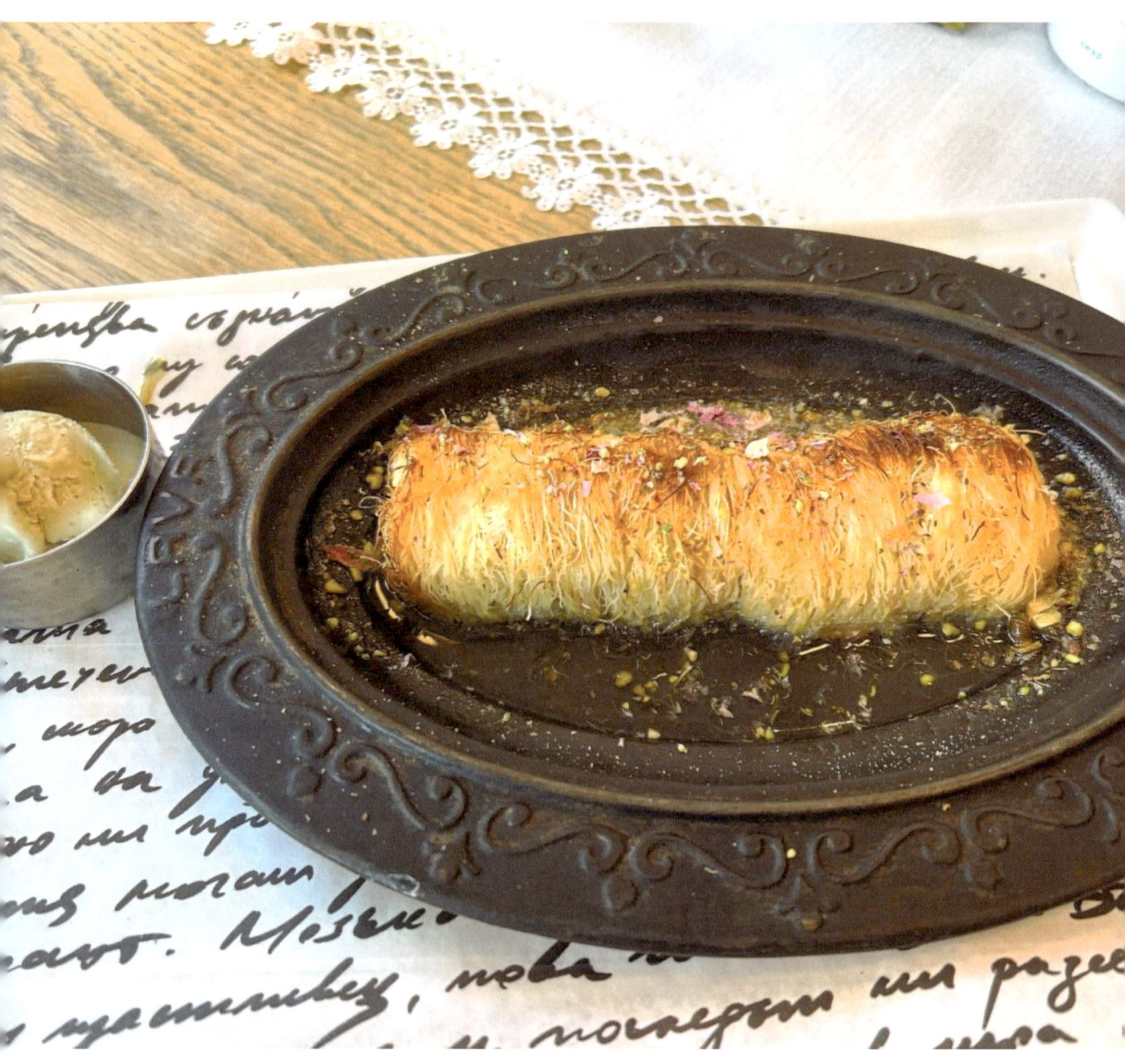

Kadaif With Cream

INGREDIENTS

    1 2/3 cup kadaif – to be found in Middle eastern or Balkan stores
    1 cup crushed walnuts
    ¾ cup butter
    ¾ cup sugar

Crème – one liter milk, 1/3 cup flour, vanilla extract, one egg yolk, 1 cup whipped cream, 1/3 cup cornmeal

The kadaif is preferably cooked first on the stove; melt the butter in a deep pan and on top place the kadaif as you pull and break it up, add the walnuts, and the sugar. Keep mixing all the time as you want the kadaif to get an even golden color. Let the kadaif cool off.

Use a mixer to mix the flour, the cornmeal, and the egg yolk, add the cold milk slowly. Then add the sugar and the vanilla extract, cook at low heat in a pot on the stove, keep mixing and when the crème thickens, add the whipped cream, stir and remove from stove. Place half of the cooled off kadaif on the bottom of the baking dish, spread all the creme on top and top with the remaining cooled off kadaif. Keep refrigerated overnight, serve cold.

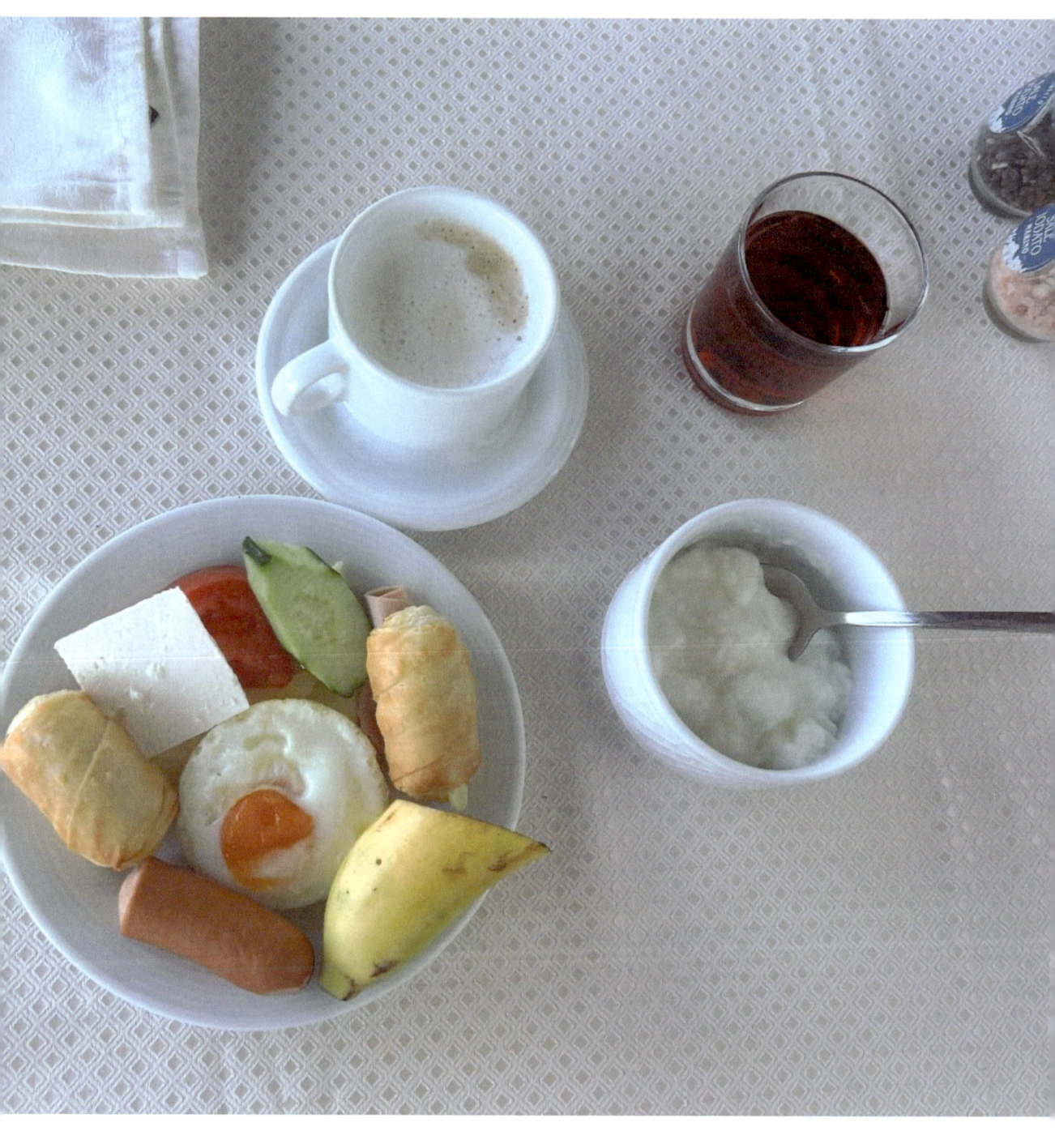

European Healthy Breakfast

A poached egg, half a banana, a couple of cucumber and tomato slices, feta cheese, banitsa bites (the Banitsa recipe is on another page of the book), half a breakfast sausage, yogurt, cappuccino, and a glass of berry juice.

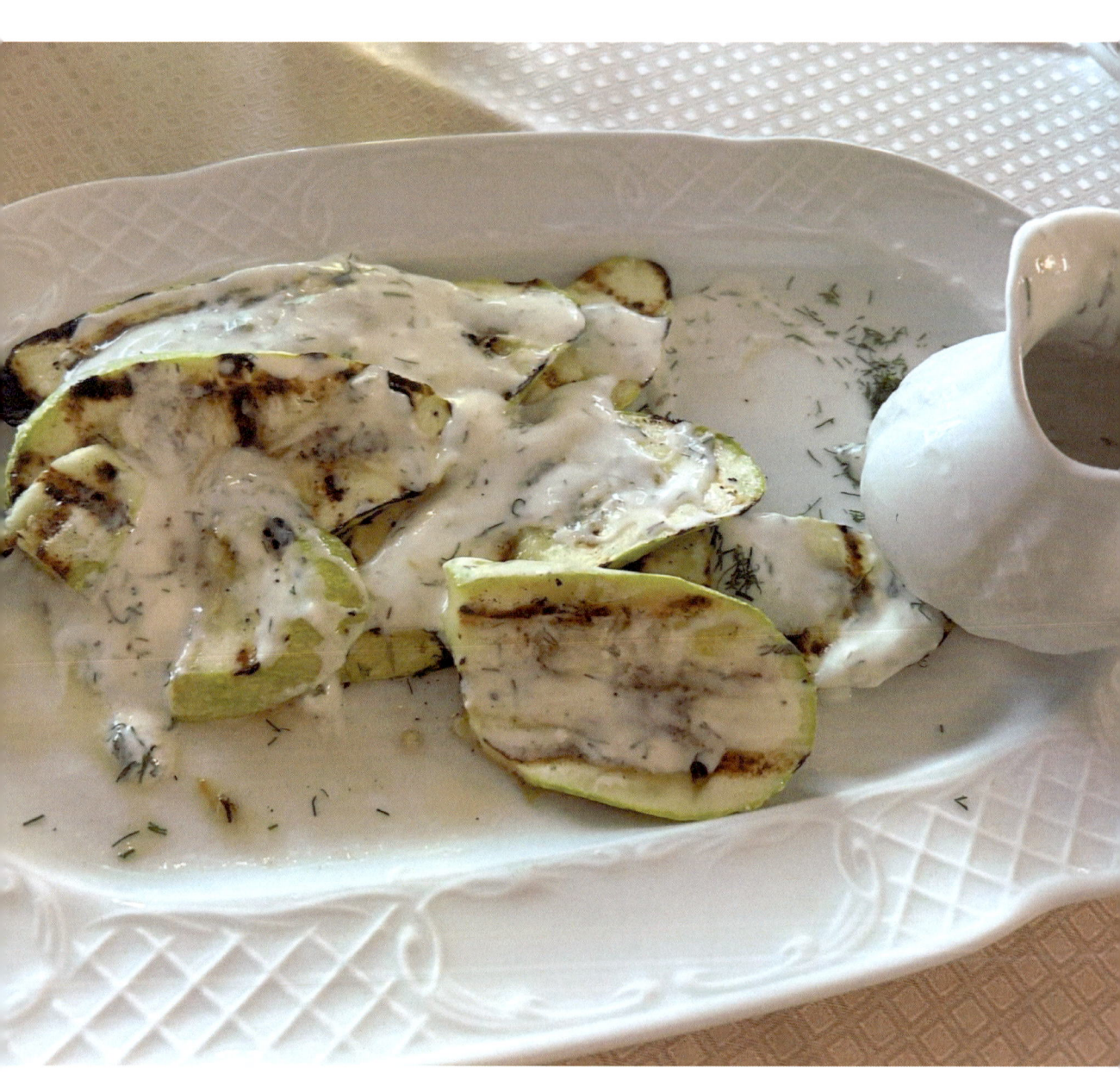

Greek Roasted Zucchini And Yogurt With Dill Sauce

INGREDIENTS

3 zucchini, olive oil, garlic, yogurt, mayo, dill, salt.

Slice the zucchini vertically in long slices ¾ of an inch wide, sprinkle with salt and smear olive oil on both sides; grill to get the color of the zucchini on the photo. For the sauce, mix two tablespoons of Greek yogurt, one tablespoon mayo, chopped dill, and 2-3 crushed garlic cloves.

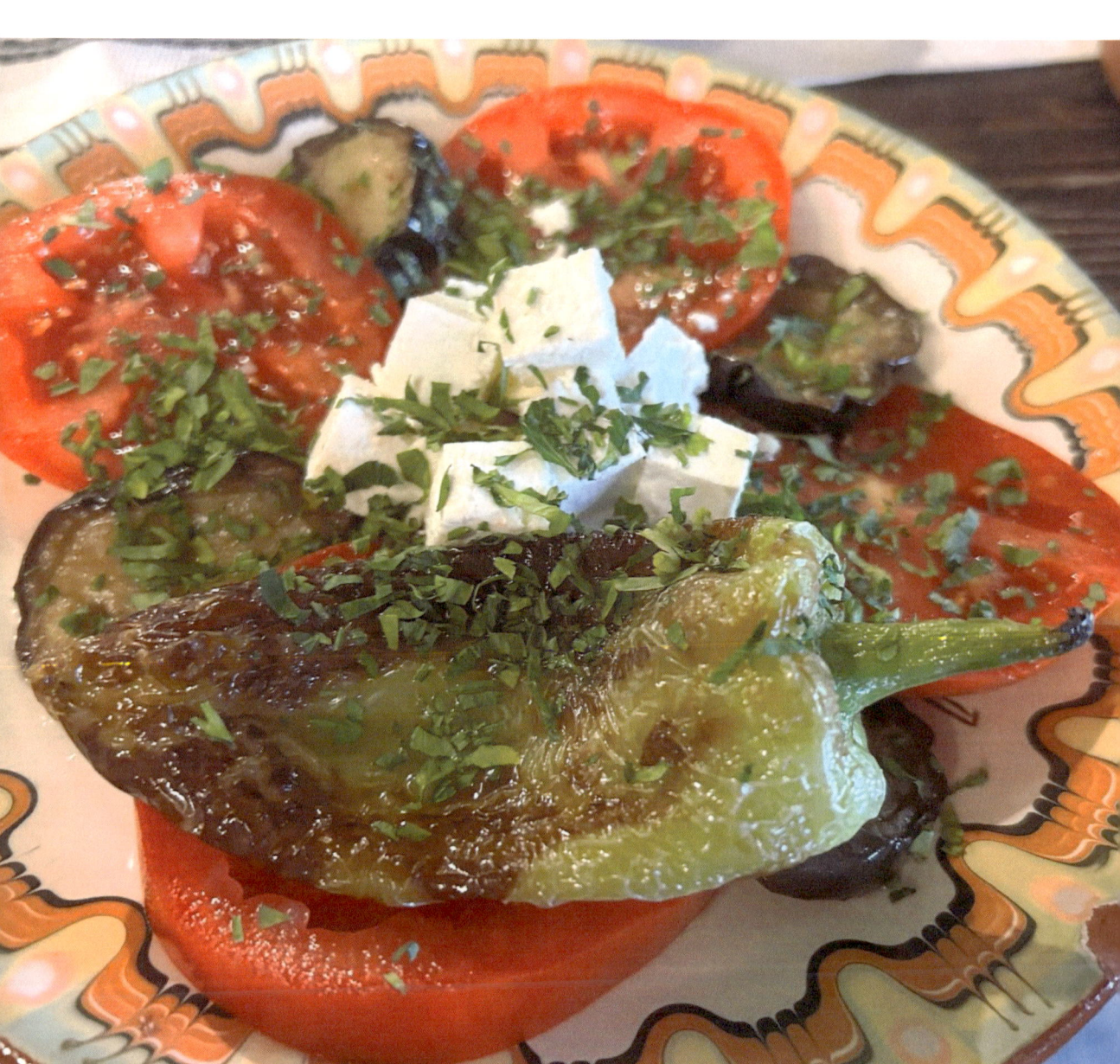

Tomato And Pepper Salad

Arrange peeled, baked green pepper and tomato slices on a serving dish, evenly pour over the mixture of salt, oil and vinegar dressing, place chunks of feta cheese on top, garnish with parsley.

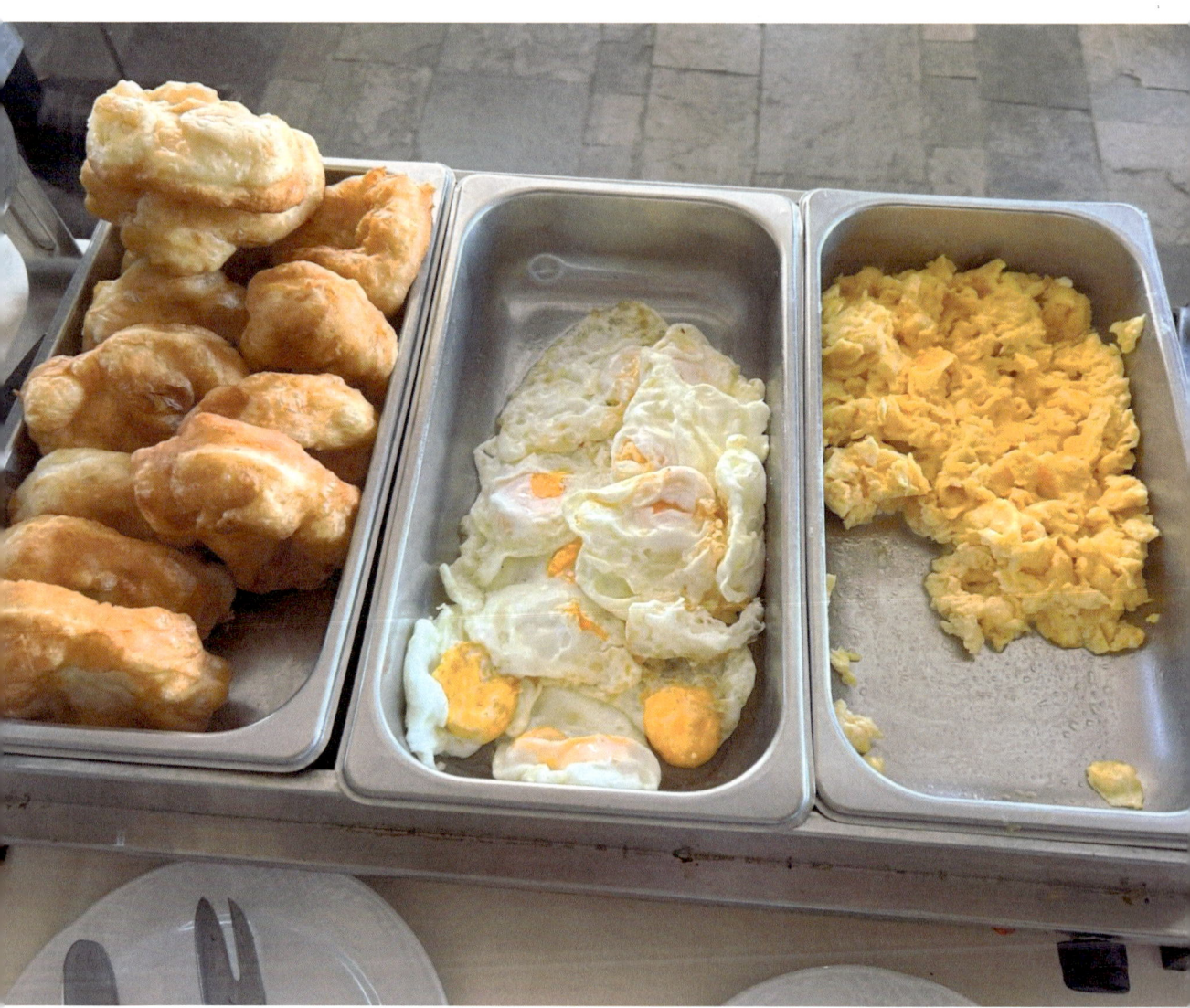

Breakfast Buffet with Ponichki (Bulgarian Donuts) Poached or Scrambled Eggs.

INGREDIENTS FOR PONICHKI

1 ¼ cups yogurt, one teaspoon baking soda, 2 eggs, 3/4 cup sugar, 3 teaspoons olive oil, one teaspoon baking powder, pinch of salt, 2 ½ cups flour, oil for cooking, powdered sugar to sprinkle on top.

Sift the flour, make a hole in the middle and pour in the yogurt, the soda, the mixed eggs, the salt, sugar, oil and baking powder. Work it to make a dough and let it rest 10-15 min. Then roll the dough, cut the rolled dough in circles, and cook in hot oil, take out when golden in color and sprinkle with powdered sugar.

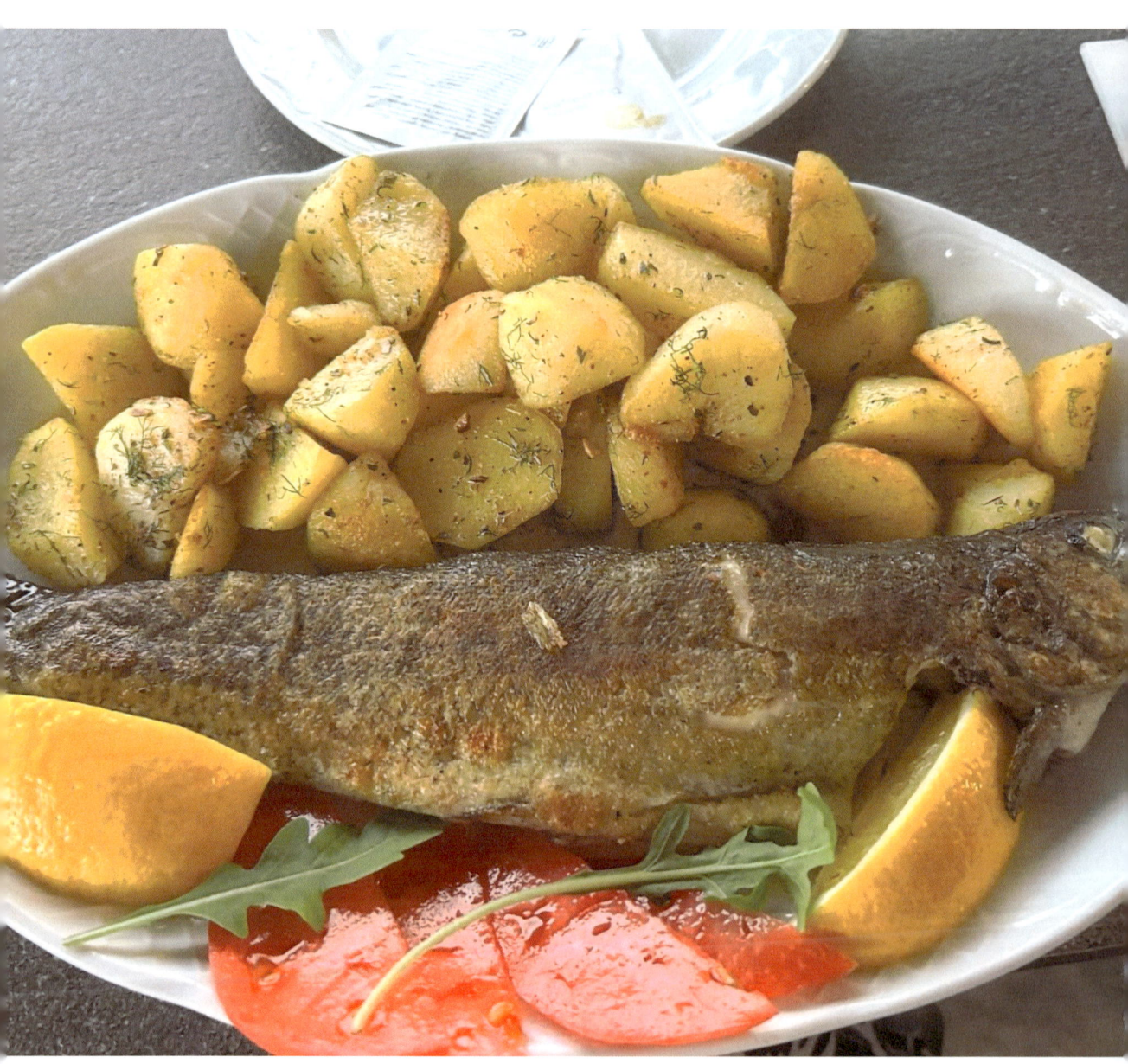

Baked Fresh Mackerel, Baked Potatoes, Slices of Tomatoes and Lemon

INGREDIENTS

Whole cleaned mackerel, sea salt, black pepper, oil, lemon, tomato, gold cut potatoes, dill.

Salt and pepper the fish, rub evenly with oil, squeeze lemon juice on top, place in a baking pan on baking paper, preheat oven to 390 degrees and bake until golden in color. Season cut potatoes with sea salt and sweet paprika and bake at 390 degrees, turning over once, until golden brown. Sprinkle with dill or parsley.

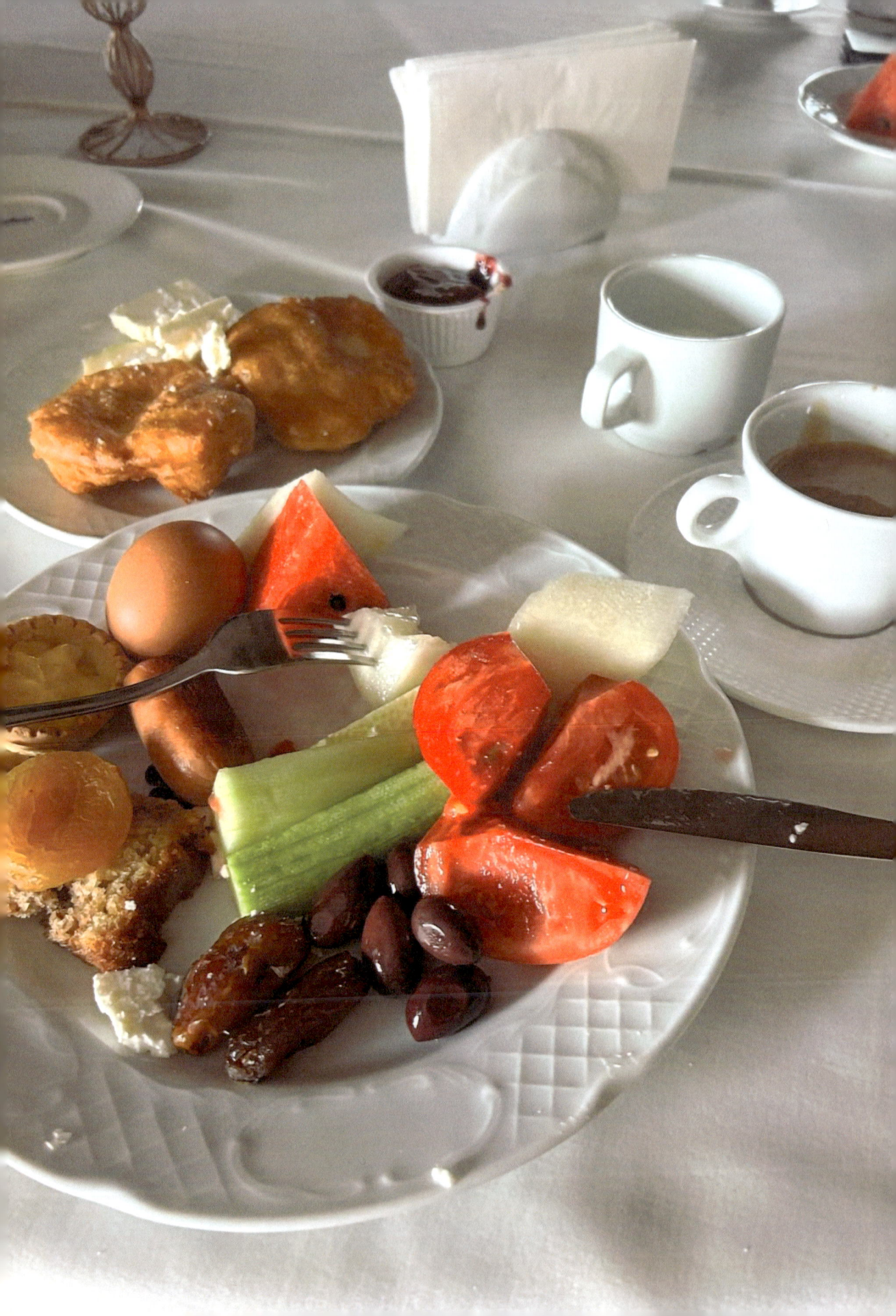

Healthy European Breakfast Buffet

Peeled and cut cucumbers, cut tomatoes in slices, slice of cut watermelon, boiled egg, olives, sausage, kashkaval (swiss cheese), piece of walnut cake, dried apricot, ponichki, cappuccino.

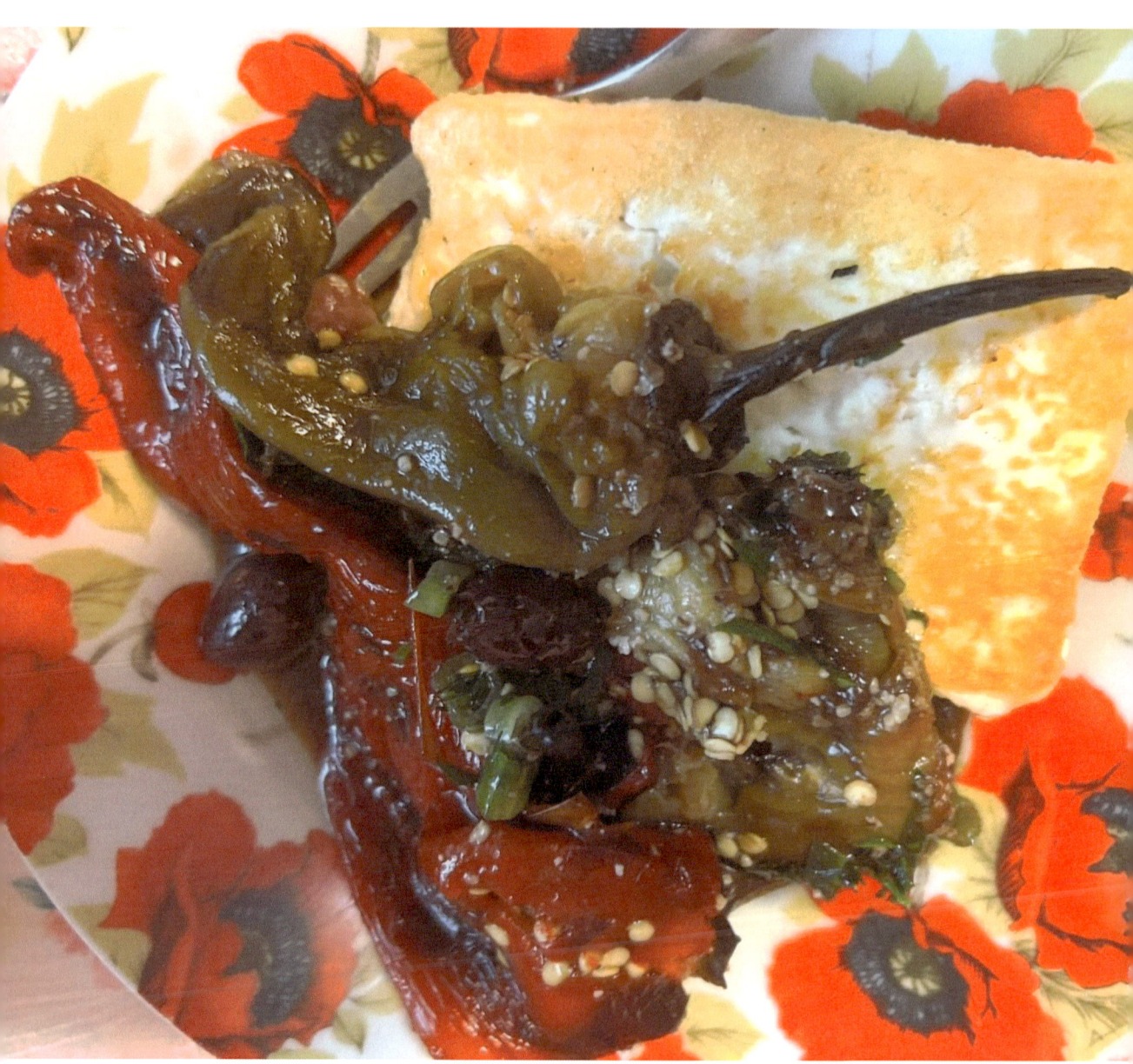

Pepper Salad and Polenta (Kachamak)

Roasted green and red long peppers, peeled with dressing of oil, vinegar, salt and crushed garlic. Slice of polenta (kachamak) – recipe on another page

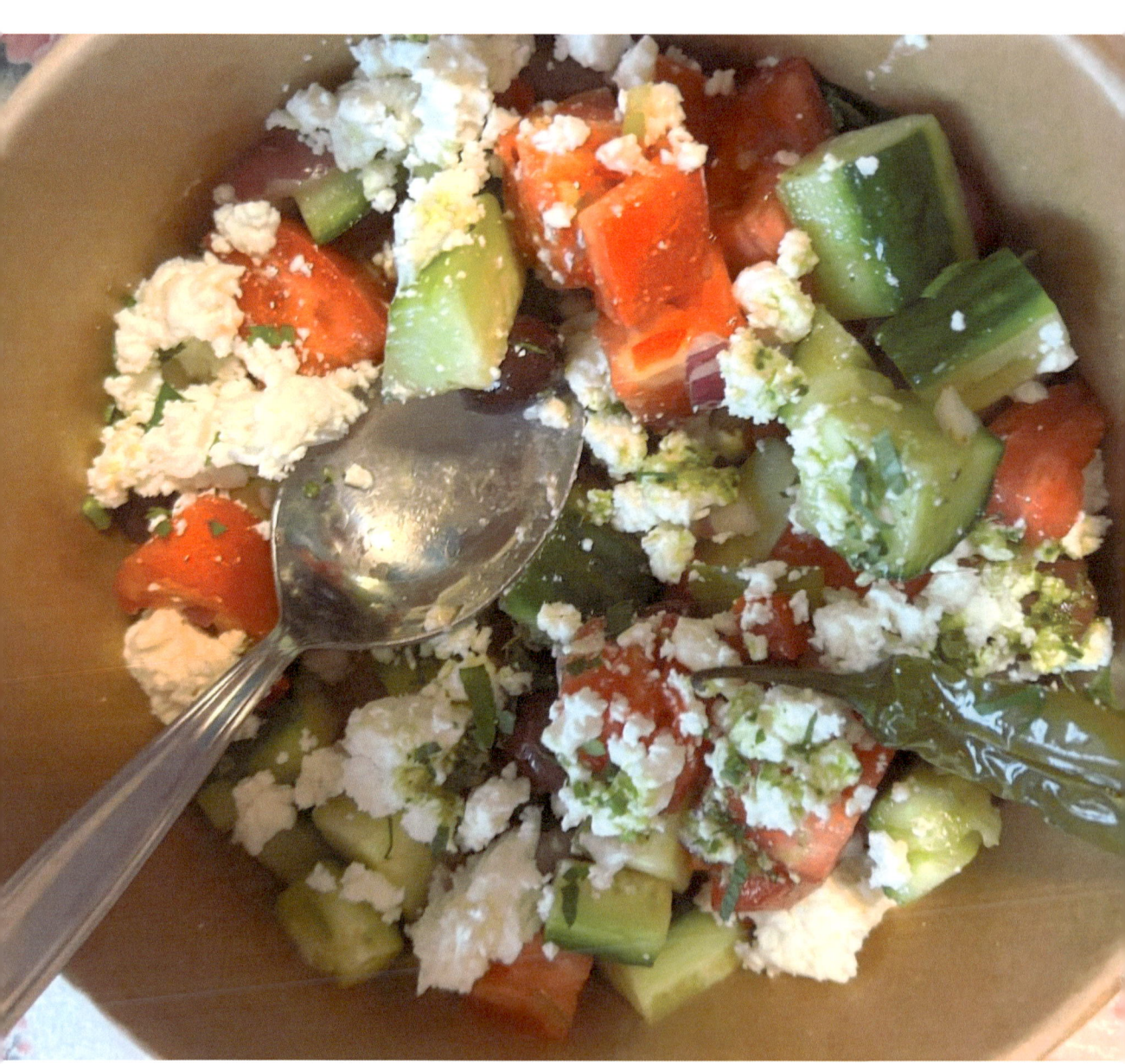

Summer Salad with Choppped Cucumbers, Cut Tomatoes, Roasted Peppers, Parsley, Feta Cheese, Oil and Vinegar Dressing.

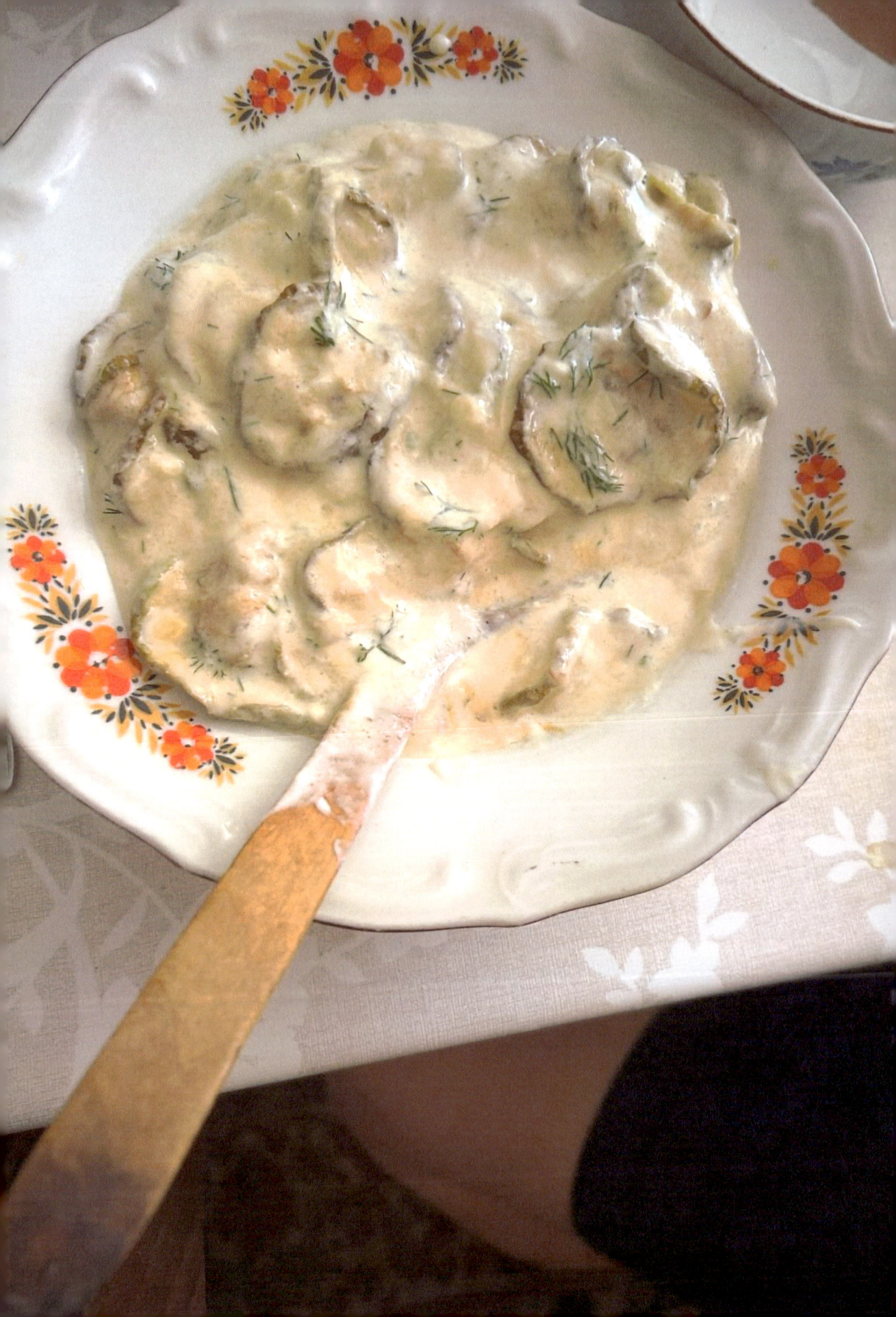

Zucchini with Yogurt, Mayo, Garlic and Dill Sauce

INGREDIENTS

Two zucchinis, thinly sliced, flour, olive oil.

Zucchini are washed and sliced thin, salted, rolled in flour and fried in a pan with hot oil. Turn over once. Sauce is same as for grilled Greek zucchini.

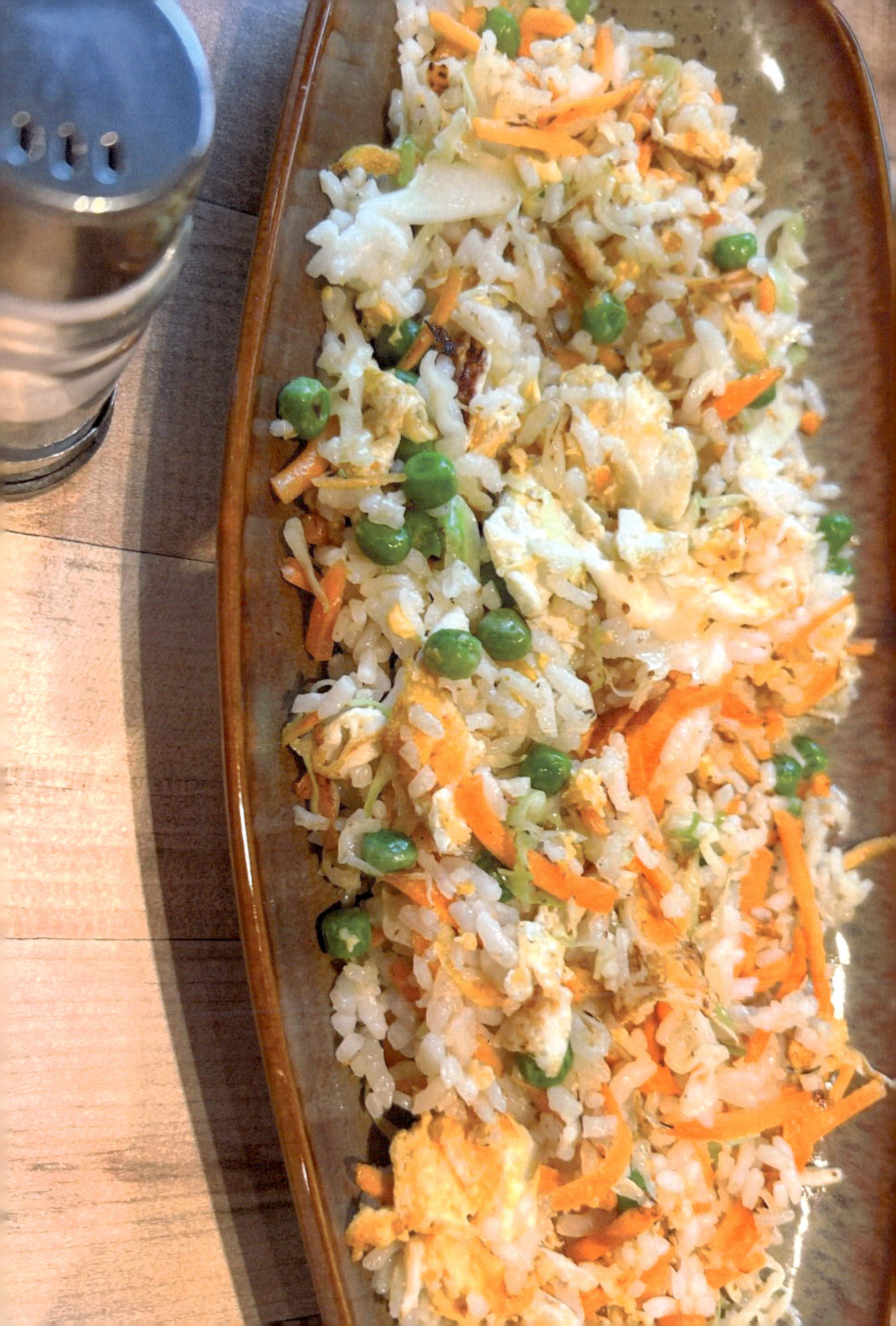

Summer Vegetarian Dish

INGREDIENTS ───────────────────────

1 cup rice, two cups vegetable broth, carrots cut in thin strips, sliced onion, peas, cauliflower florets cut in half, soup spoon of olive oil, chubritsa or Italian seasoning, salt and pepper.

Mix all ingredients except peas, place in a baking dish, cover with aluminum foil and bake at 400 degrees for half an hour, remove foil and stir in peas, bake again for 5 minutes. Ovens are different, taste the rice to see if it is fully cooked.

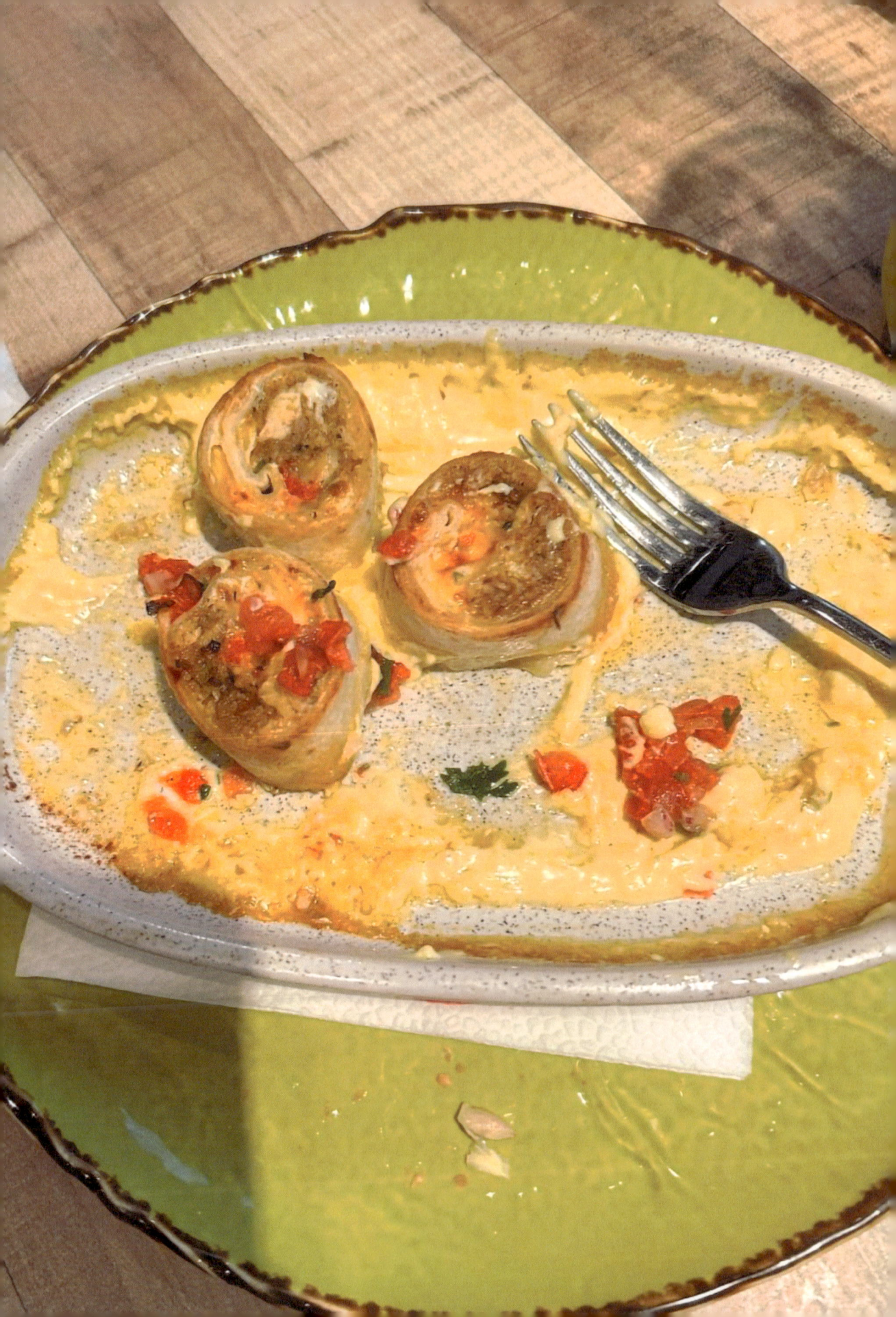

Baked Vegetables Topped with Mozarella and Yellow Cheeses Garnished with Stuffed Mushrooms

INGREDIENTS

Red, green and orange peppers, onion, garlic, tomatoes, carrots, celery, ½ cup of rice, cup and a half vegetable broth, tablespoon of olive oil, mushrooms without stems and stuffed with chorizo and chopped tomato, Italian seasoning or chubritsa, vegeta seasoning (can be found in Balkan and Arabic food stores), or salt and black pepper, mozzarella and yellow cheeses.

Chop and cut vegetables to your liking, mix vegetables with oil, rice, add spices, vegetable broth, olive oil, vegeta and place in a clay pot. Cook for half an hour at 390 degrees, then uncover and sprinkle with mozzarella and unevenly with yellow cheese, top with mushrooms stuffed with chorizo and chopped tomato, return to oven for 10 min.

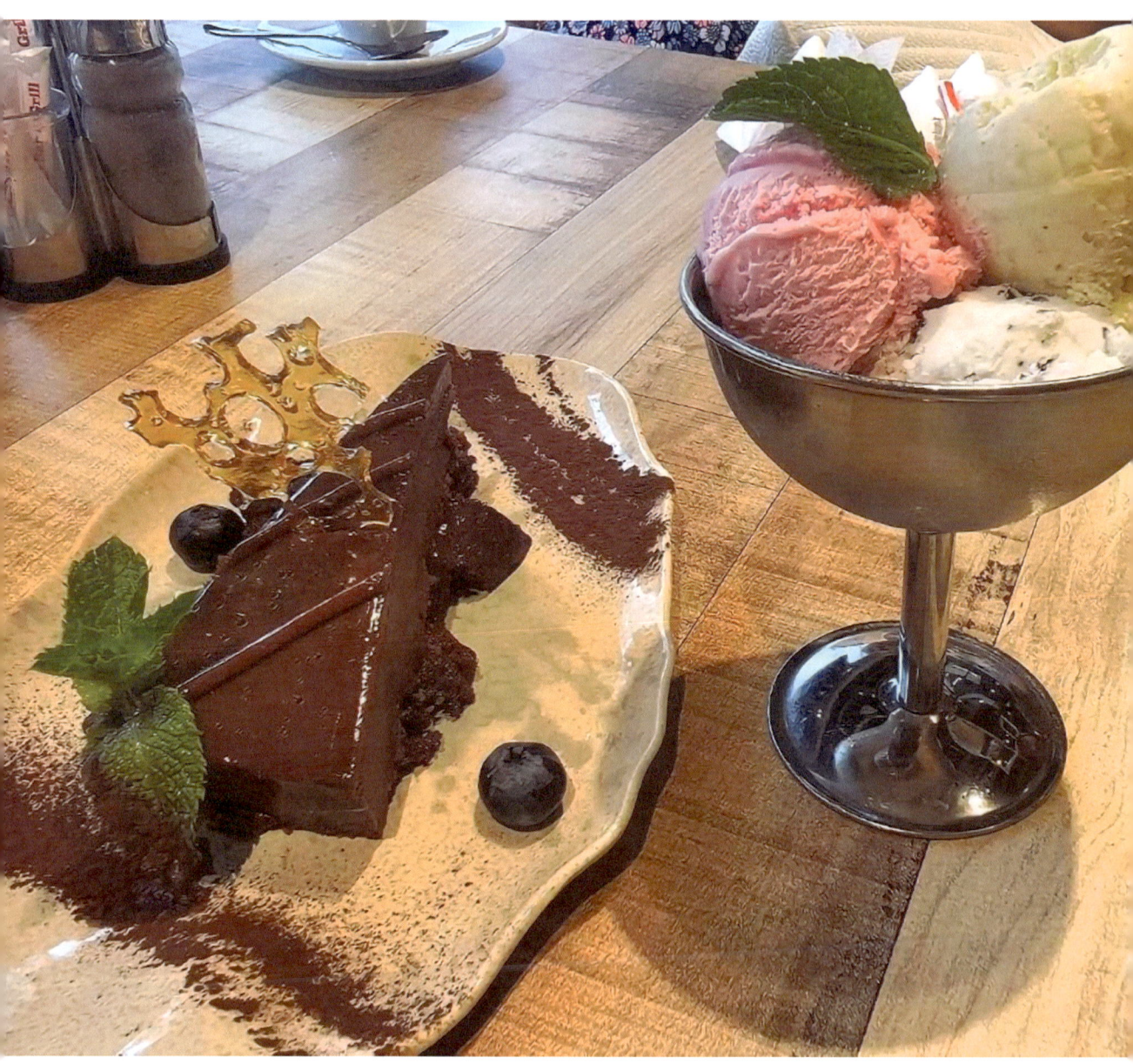

Deserts Delight - Chocolate Cake, Three Kinds of Icecream

INGREDIENTS CHOCOLATE CAKE ——————

One cup of flour, package of baking powder, 1 1/3 cup sugar, ½ cup cocoa, 4 eggs, 200 ml milk, ½ cup avocado oil, finely chopped walnuts.

FOR THE CRÈAM: 200 grams of black chocolate, 1 cup butter, whipped cream.

Mix half of the ingredients of the flour, cocoa, baking powder and sugar in a bowl, beat the eggs separately, Add half of the milk to the bowl, half the oil, walnuts, mix well and add 2 eggs.

Pour the mixed dough on a baking dish previously dusted with flour and bake 20 min.at 370 degrees. Prepare the second layer in the same way. Let the layers cool off.

For the cream, melt the butter and the chocolate pieces to mix well but do not boil the mixture, let the chocolate mixture cool off a little and add the whipped cream. Use this chocolate mixture to connect the two layers. Spread on top the remaining cream. Ice cream is purchased per your choice.

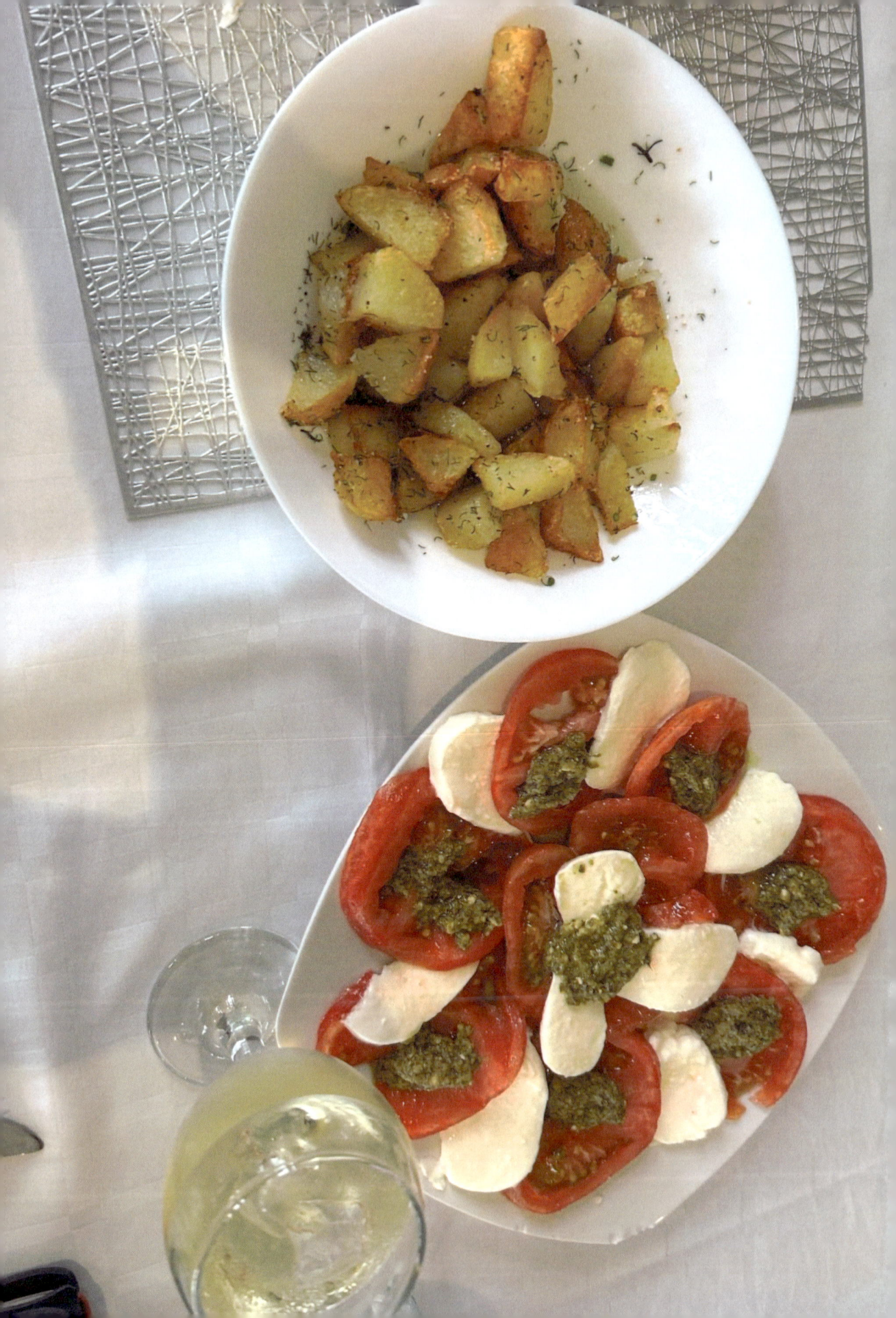

Simple Light Lunch

INGREDIENTS

Yellow potatoes, tomato slices, fresh mozzarella cheese, garlic basil spread (basil leaves, garlic, oil and salt are mixed in a blender). Accompanied by a glass of chilled white wine or grape juice.

Potatoes are cut, seasoned with sea salt and sweet red paprika, mixed with oil and baked at 390 degrees, sprinkled with dill for serving.

Arrange the sliced tomatoes and mozzarella cheese on a serving dish, spread the basil garlic on top of the tomato slices and cheese as shown on the photo, add olives if you wish.

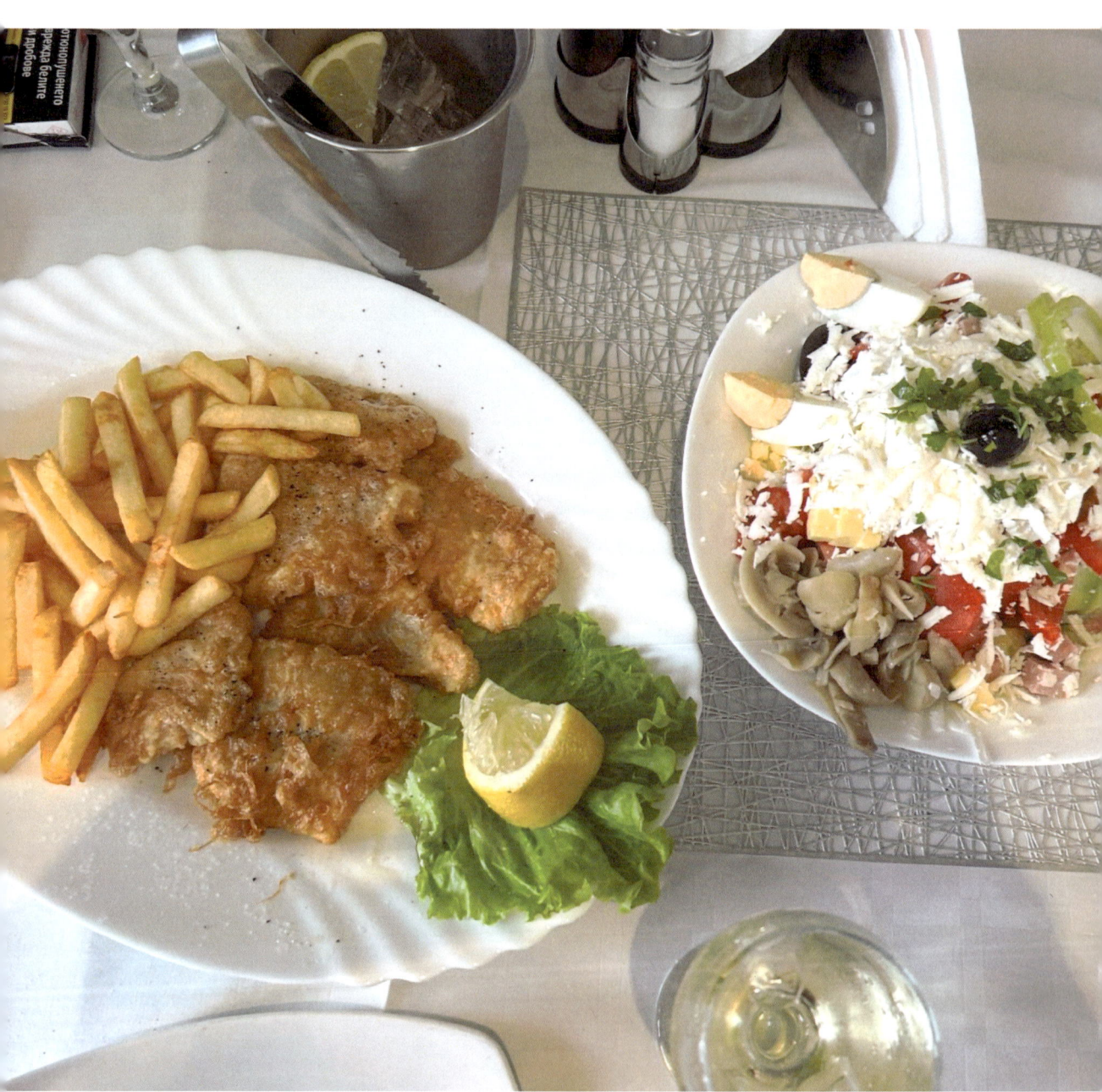

Schnitzel with Fried Potatoes, Lemon Slice and Lettuce Leaf. Shepherd's Salad.

INGREDIENTS

150 grams of veal fillet, salt, ¼ cup of flour, one egg, ¼ cup of breadcrumbs, olive oil.

Pound the meat and make cuts on the edges with a sharp knife. Roll the fillet first in flour, shake off the excess flour, then dip in the egg and then the breadcrumbs. Heat 2 cm of oil in a pan and fry on both sides, from time to time shake the pan to allow the oil to cover the schnitzel. Place the cooked schnitzel on a paper towel to absorb the oil and serve with side dishes of your choice – vegetables or French fries as on this photo.

Shepherd's Salad

Two tomatoes, cucumber, two baked and peeled peppers, ¼ red onion, 100 g marinated mushrooms, grated feta cheese, 120 g finely cut ham, kaskaval (yellow cheese), two hard-boiled eggs, two soup spoons of olive oil, vinegar, parsley, salt, olives.

Cut the tomatoes, cucumber and peppers, then cut the onion into half-moon slices, arrange them in a bowl with the mushrooms, ham, and cheese cut in cubes. Sprinkle the grated feta cheese on top, decorate with the sliced eggs, and the olives, garnish with parsley.

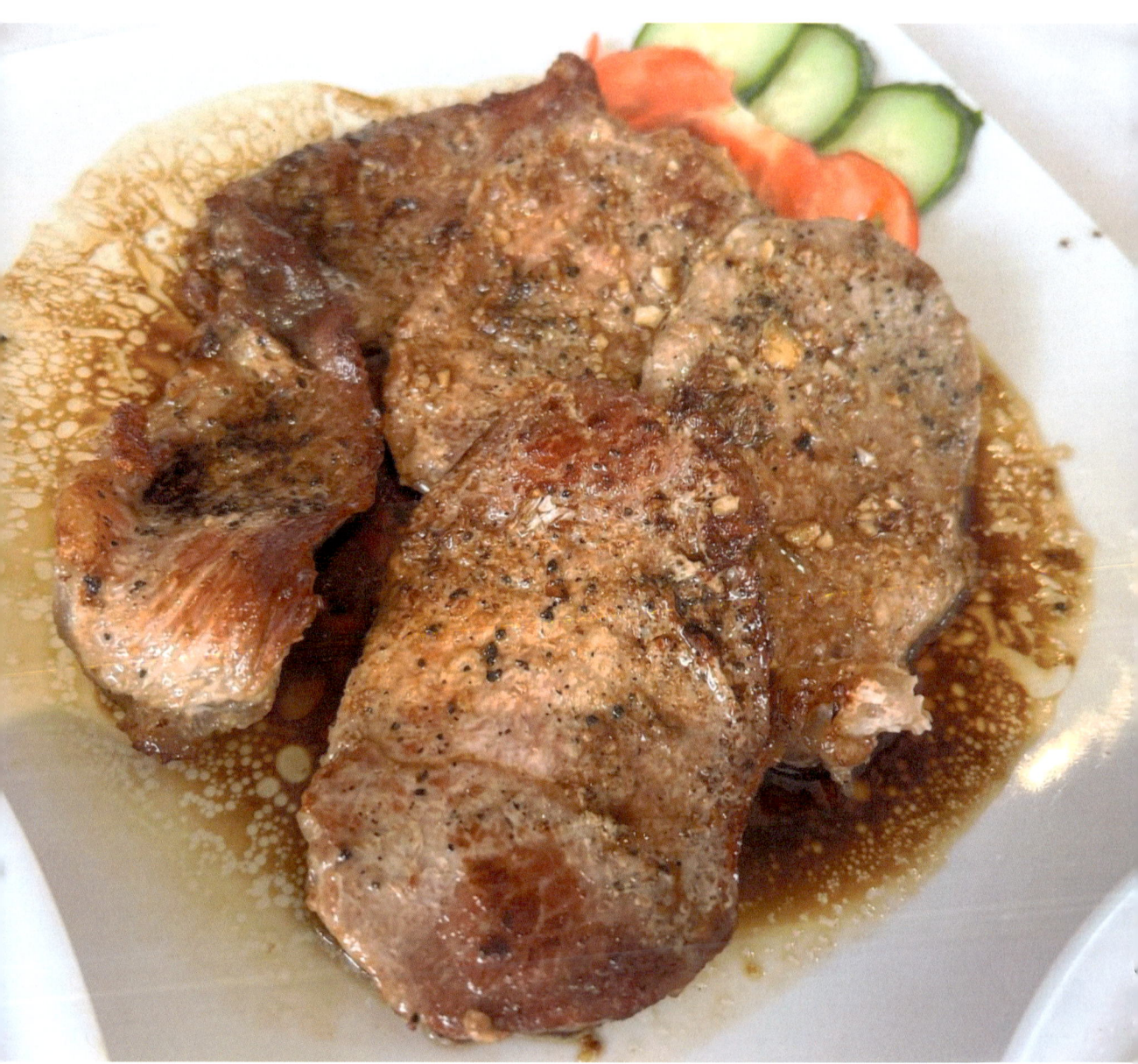

Veal or Pork Baked Shank

INGREDIENTS

Veal or pork shank, garlic, onion, red wine, soy sauce, vegetable broth, peppercorn, sweet paprika, olive oil, Italian seasoning or chubritsa, bay leaves

Make openings in the meat for garlic and peppercorn and stuff with pieces of garlic and peppercorns, place the shanks in a clay pot, combine in a dish a cup of red wine, minced garlic, a tablespoon of soy sauce and olive oil, paprika, Italian seasoning, finely diced head of onion, rub into the meat and pour the remaining liquid into the pot, add two cups of vegetable broth, place in the oven at 420 degrees. Bake for an hour, remove from the oven if the meat is tender when checked with thermometer.

Make a sauce by mixing the remaining liquid with a spoon of flour (teaspoon or tablespoon depending on the amount of liquid left in the pot), place on stove for a minute to thicken. Serve with slices of cucumber and tomato and rice on the side. Rice recipes can be made with mushrooms and olives.

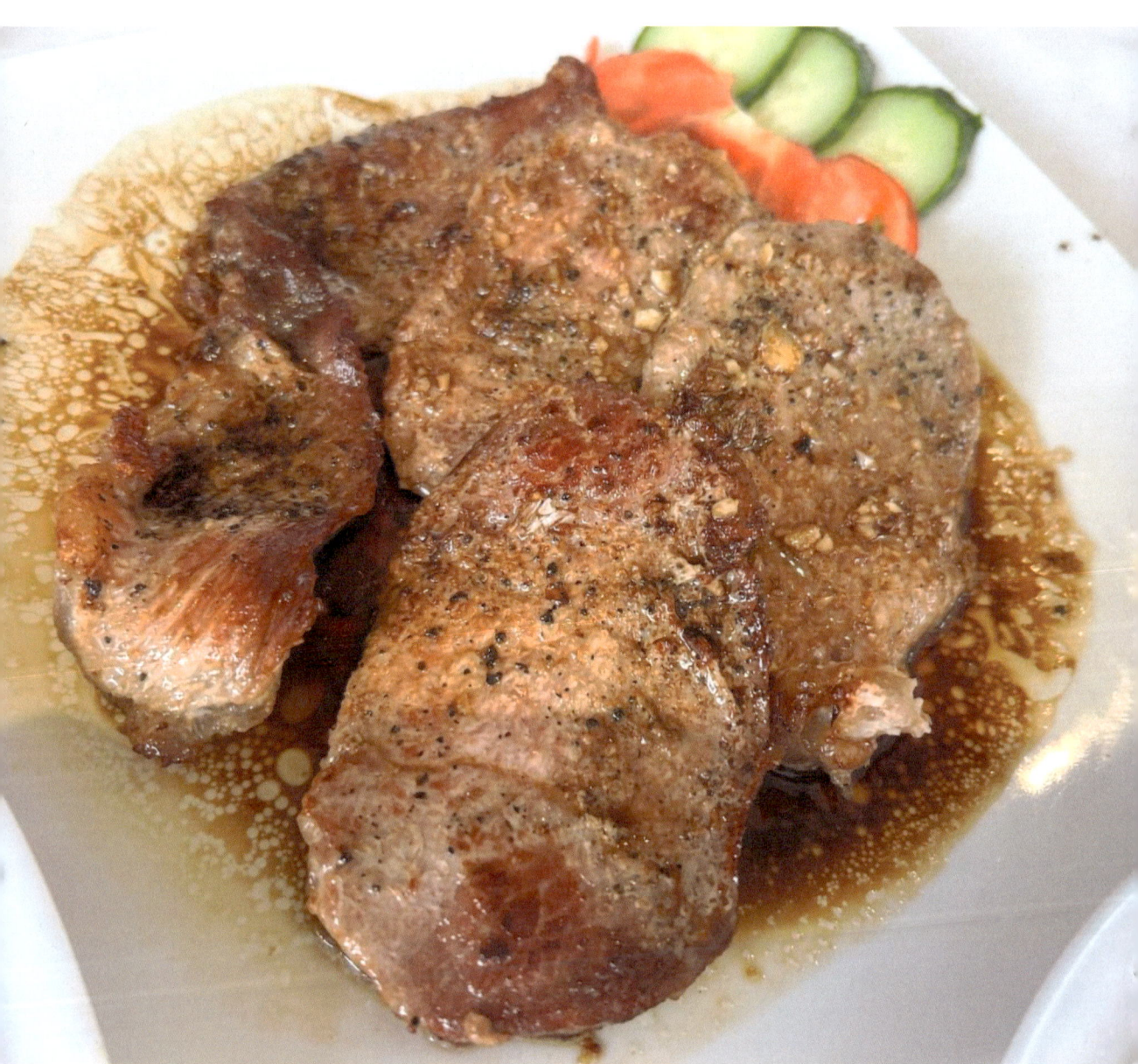

Simple Rice Recipe Ingredients

1 ½ cup mushrooms, 1 cup of rice, one small onion, half a stick of butter, 2 ¼ cups warm water, 1/2 cup mushroom gravy, parsley, black pepper, turmeric, salt.

Melt the butter in a pan, add and simmer the minced onion on medium to low heat for 5 minutes, add the cut mushrooms, then the rice, mix until the rice has a yellowish color, stir the mushroom gravy with the water and add to the pan, cook on medium to low heat for 10-15 minutes with a covered lid. As soon as the rice absorbs the water add chopped parsley, sprinkle with black pepper, turmeric powder, and teaspoon of salt (as per your taste). Take off the stove and leave for 10 minutes with the lid on before serving.

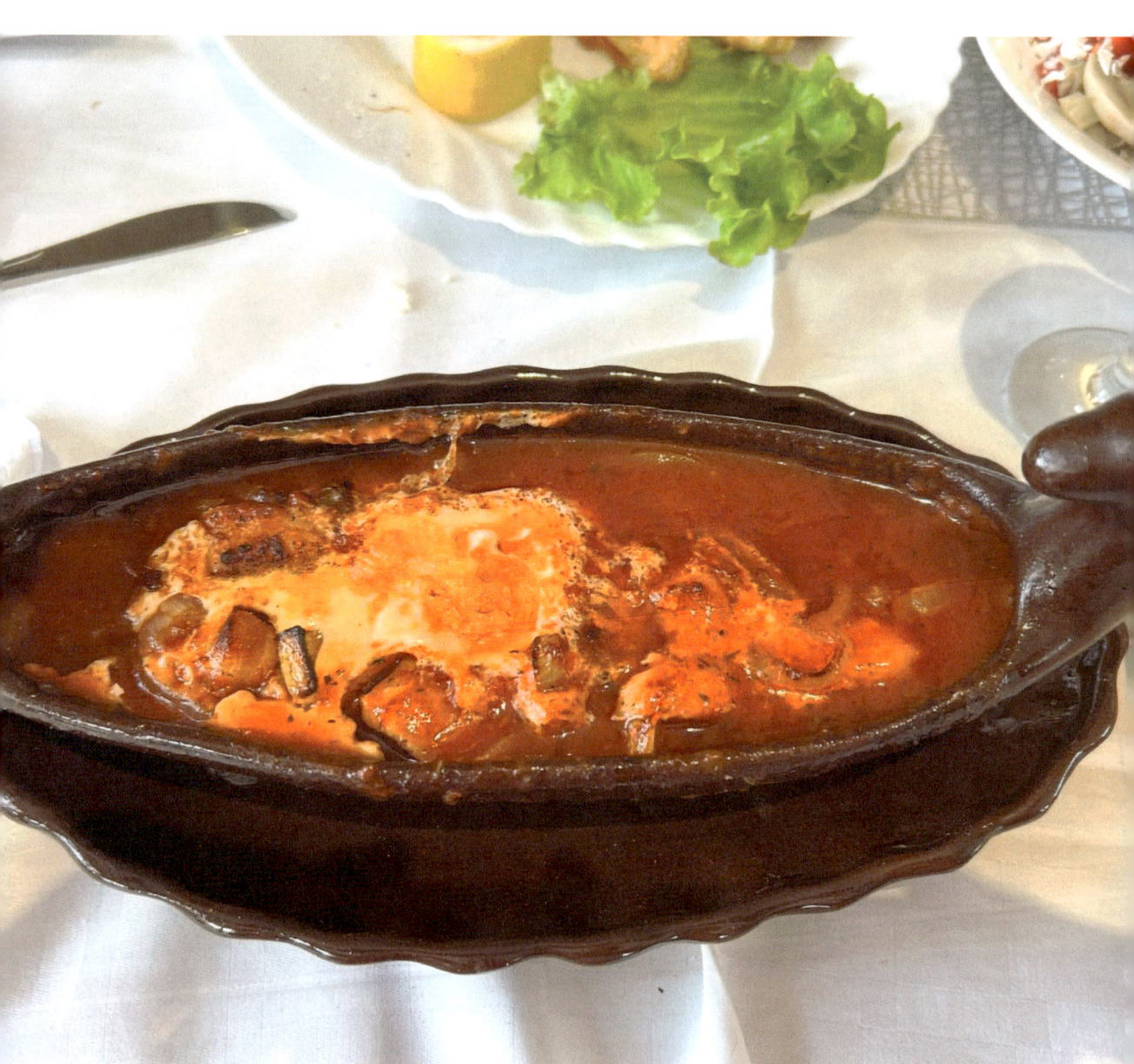

Baked Vegetables and Cheese in Individual Clay Pot

INGREDIENTS

150-200 grams of feta cheese, 100 grams lukanka or hard salami, one onion, two baked and peeled red peppers, 100-150 grams tomato juice, 50 grams butter, one egg, sweet paprika, black pepper, parsley, one tomato.

Smear the butter all over the inner side of the clay pot, on the bottom, place half of the cut onion and one pepper, then the cheese and the lukanka or salami cut in cubes, add the remaining onion and pepper, pour over the tomato juice, and add on top the sliced tomato, break the egg (do not mix) on top, sprinkle with sweet paprika and black pepper. Cover with a lid and bake for 15-20 min. at 290 degrees. Take out of the oven, leave covered for about 10 min. sprinkle with parsley before serving.

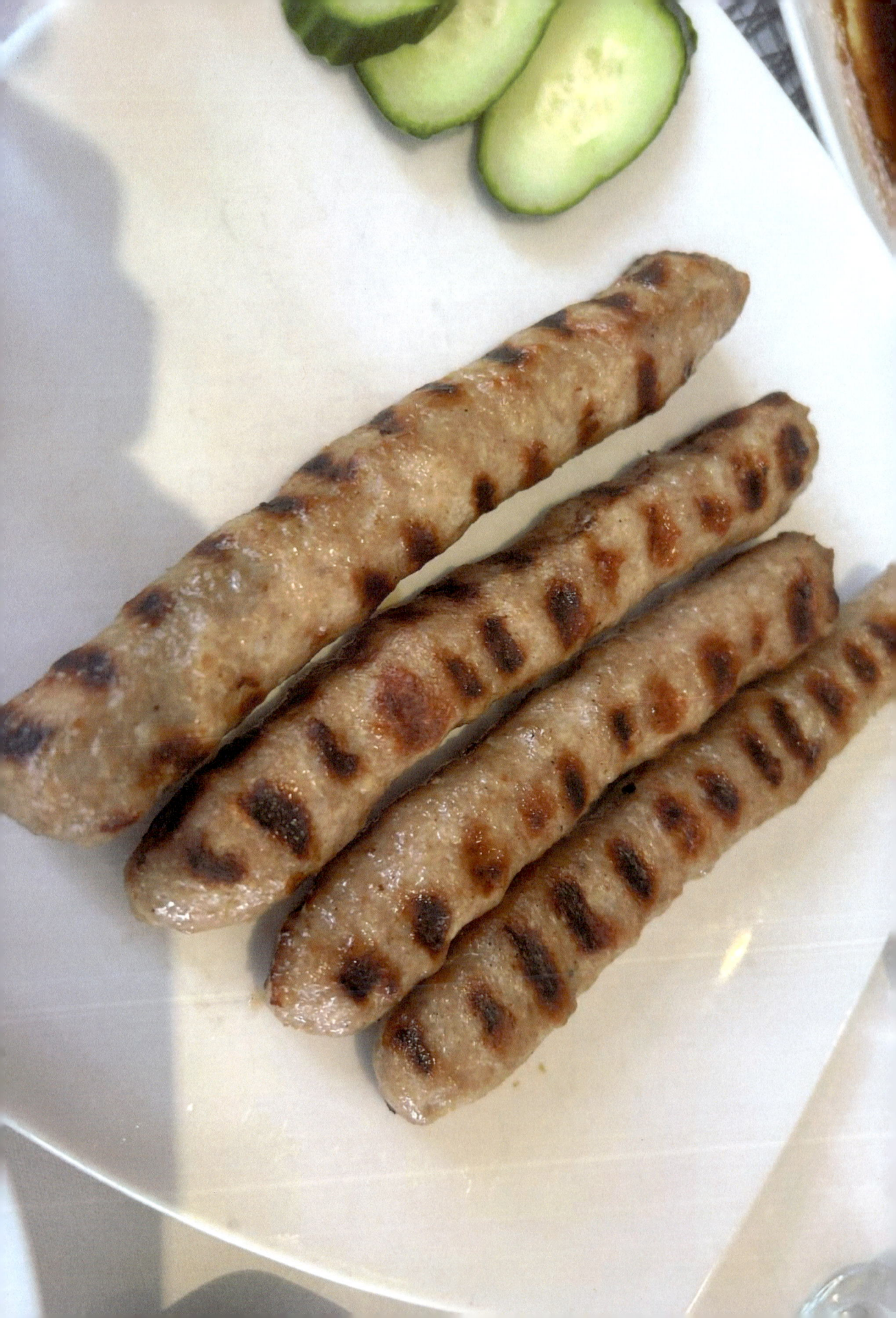

Grilled Kebapcheta - Bulgarian Recipe

INGREDIENTS

1 kg ground beef and pork – 40/60, one teaspoon cumin, 1/3 teaspoon baking soda, one or two teaspoons of salt, black pepper, 200 ml carbonated water or beer

Mix all ingredients well with 100 ml carbonated water or beer, let the mixture rest overnight, then add the remaining 100 ml of liquid and mix well again, form the kebapcheta as shown on the photo and grill on slightly greased grill on high. Serve with summer salad (tomatoes, cucumbers, red onion, olives, feta cheese, parsley and vinaigrette dressing), or green salad (lettuce, radishes, fresh onion and vinaigrette dressing).

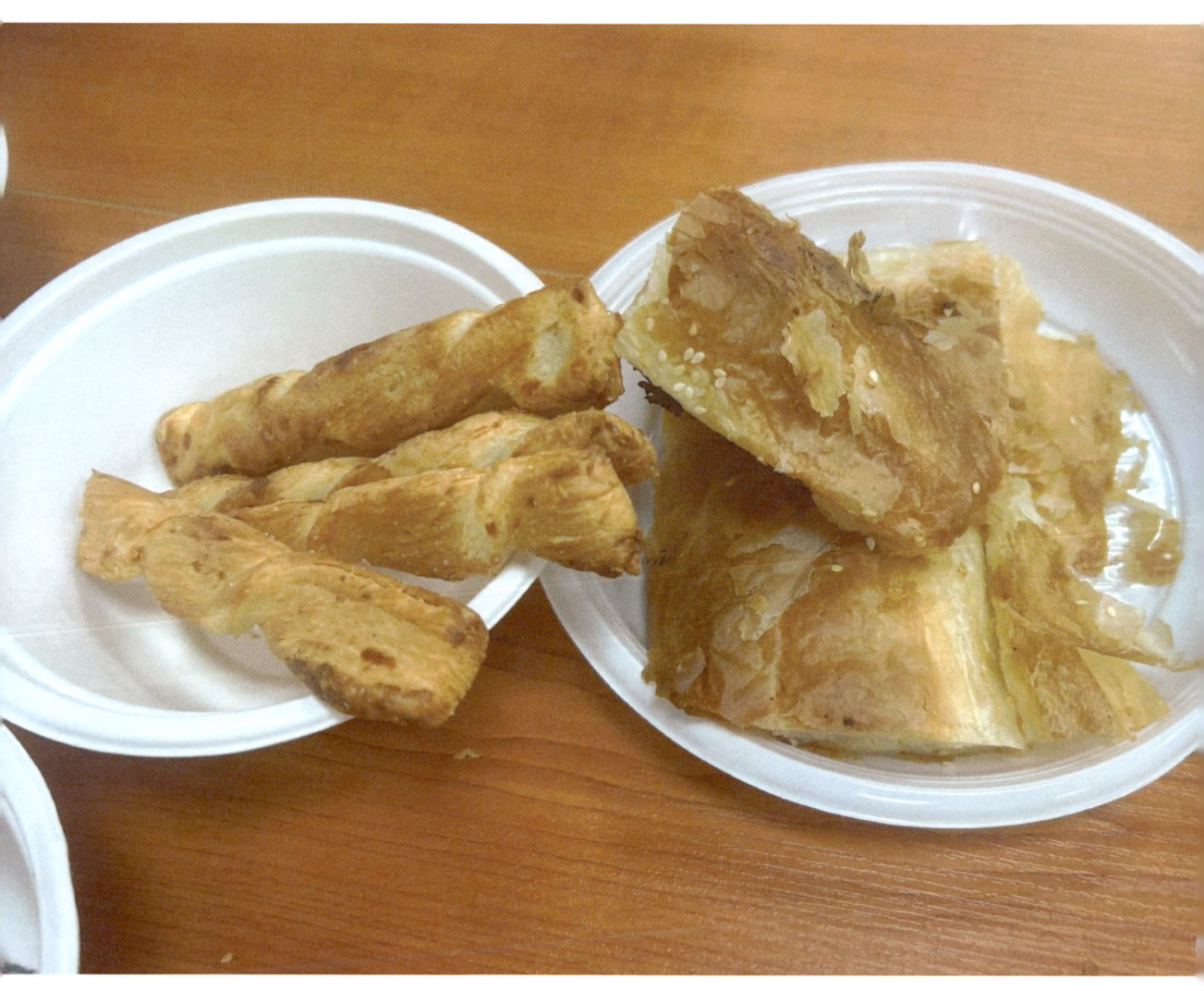

Bulgarian Breakfast on The Run - Slices of Banitsa and Cheese Sticks of Dough and Cheese.

The recipe will be provided on another page. Suggested drink is Airan, yogurt drink.

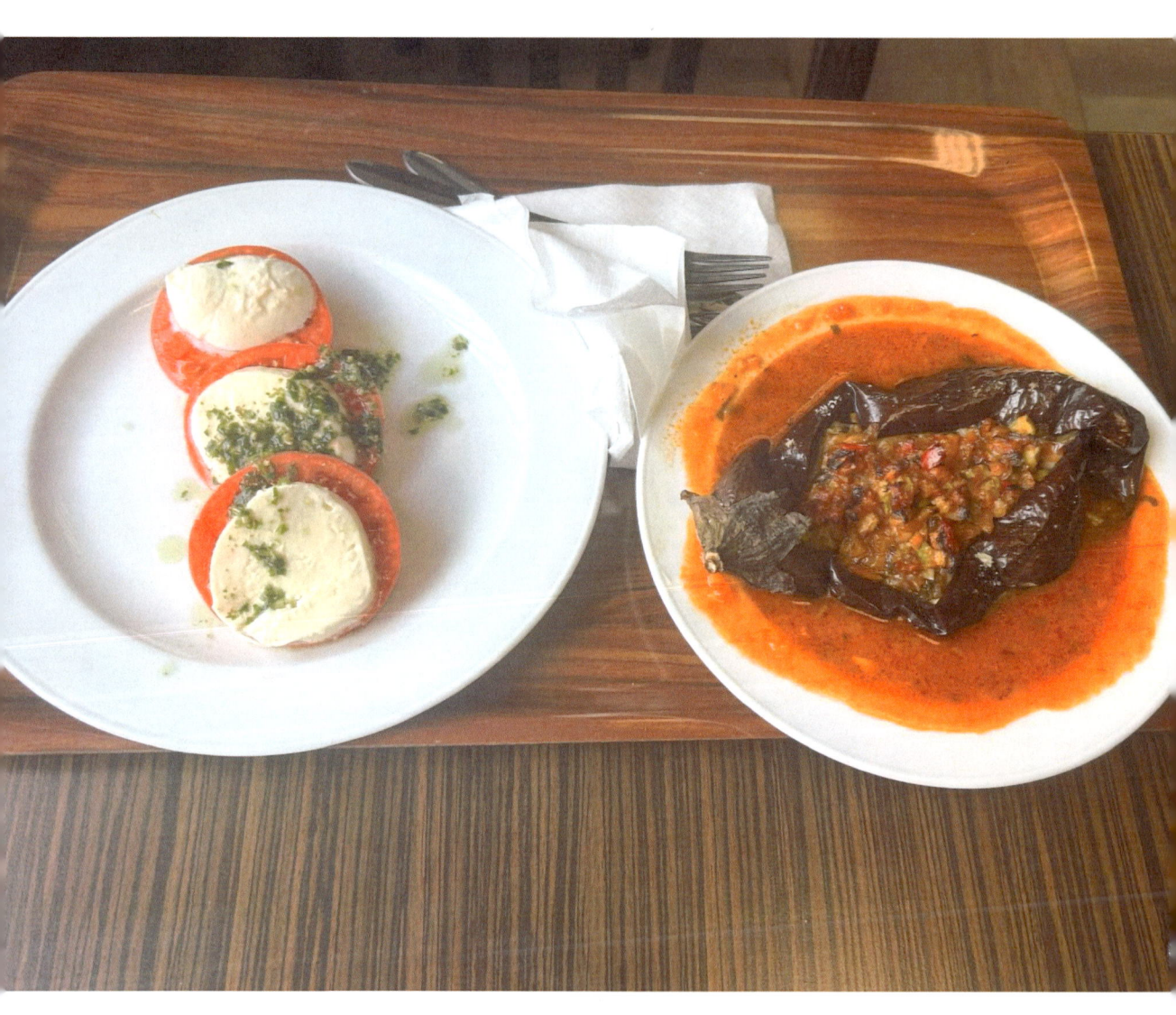

Stuffed Eggplant with Vegetables, Salad of Tomatoes and Slices of Fresh Mozzarella.

INGREDIENTS

Two eggplants, one sweet onion, two carrots, one red and green peppers, three tomatoes, 5 cloves of garlic, bay leaf, salt and black pepper, sweet paprika, parsley, 1 ½ cups vegetable broth, tomato or spaghetti sauce, ½ cup of rice, olive oil.

Cut the eggplants in half and scoop out the inside of the eggplants, salt the inside and let them rest for half an hour.

Simmer the onion, the thinly sliced carrots, the cut peppers, tomatoes, and the garlic for 10 min., add the rice and 1/1/2 cup of vegetable broth, add the spices, stir and cook with the lid on for 20 minutes

The rice should be soft.

Cover the bottom of a baking dish with tomato or spaghetti sauce. Place the eggplants in the baking dish and bake for 10-15 min. at 390 degrees. Take out of the oven and fill the eggplants with the vegetable and rice mixture, pour half a cup of vegetable broth over them and bake for another 15 min. Sprinkle with parsley before serving.

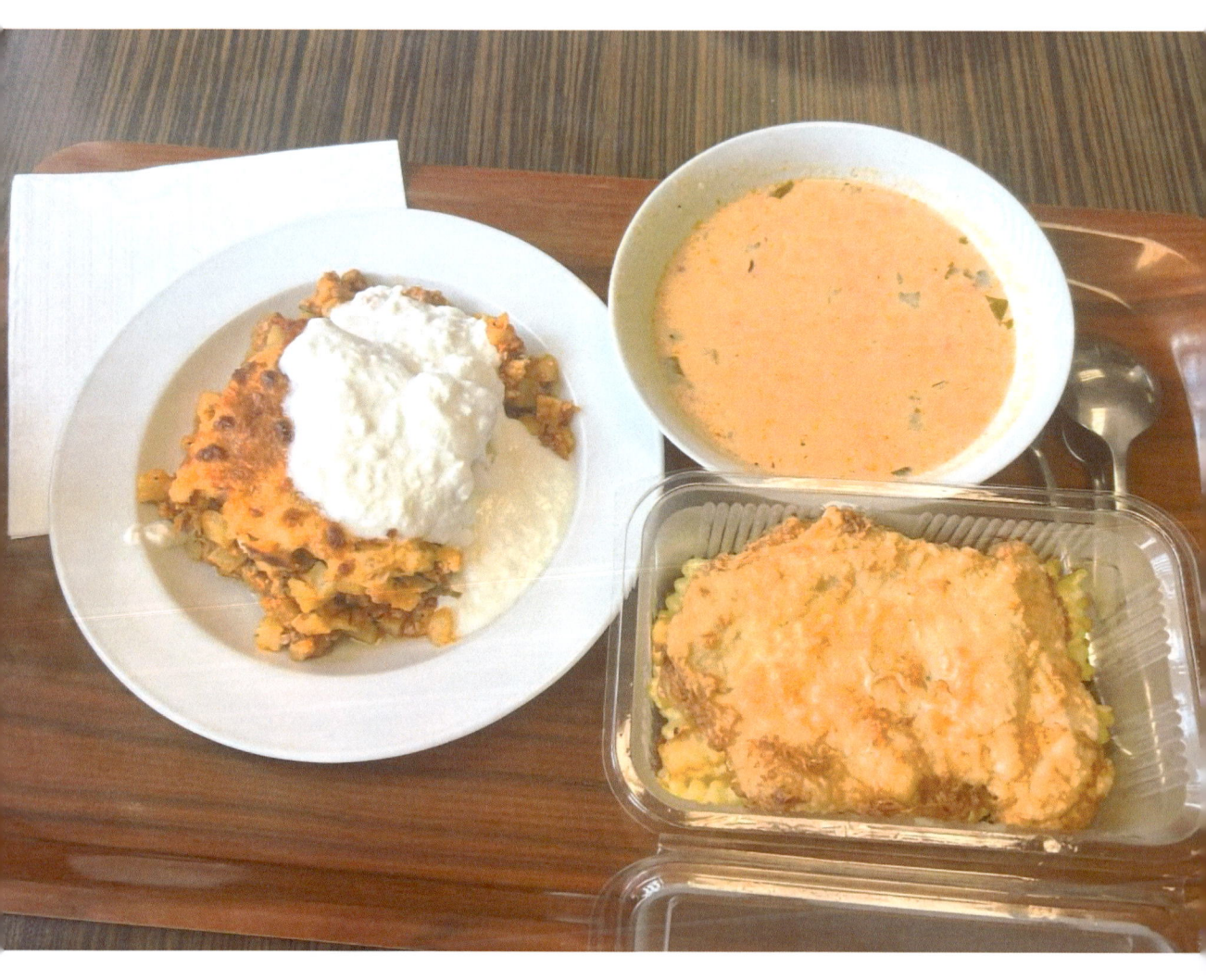

Lunch Menu

MEATBALL SOUP, MOUSSAKA, SCHNITZEL -

Meatball Soup

INGREDIENTS

½ pound of ground beef or lamb, ½ cup of rice, spices – salt, black pepper, turmeric, cumin, cardamon, coriander, carrot, celery, one onion, two potatoes, one red pepper, noodles, two cups vegetable broth, two eggs, three tablespoons yogurt, teaspoon vinegar.

Sauté the chopped onion in a pot, add the grated carrot and the cut pepper, cover and cook until the veggies are semi soft. Add the potatoes cut in cubes, the celery cut in pieces, mix well and add 1 1/2 cup vegetable stock, add salt and black pepper and cook until the mixture starts boiling.

In a bowl, mix the ground beef with the spices, salt, and ½ of parsley, mix in the rice and refrigerate for 15 min. then form small balls from the meat mixture and when the soup starts boiling add the meat balls and the soup noodles. The soup is done when the meat balls appear on the surface.

In a separate bowl, mix the yogurt, eggs and vinegar. Use a soup ladle to take some of the soup, let it cool off and mix it well in the soup, continue until the yogurt and egg mixture is mixed well with all the soup. Move the pot from the stove, mix again and sprinkle with parsley.

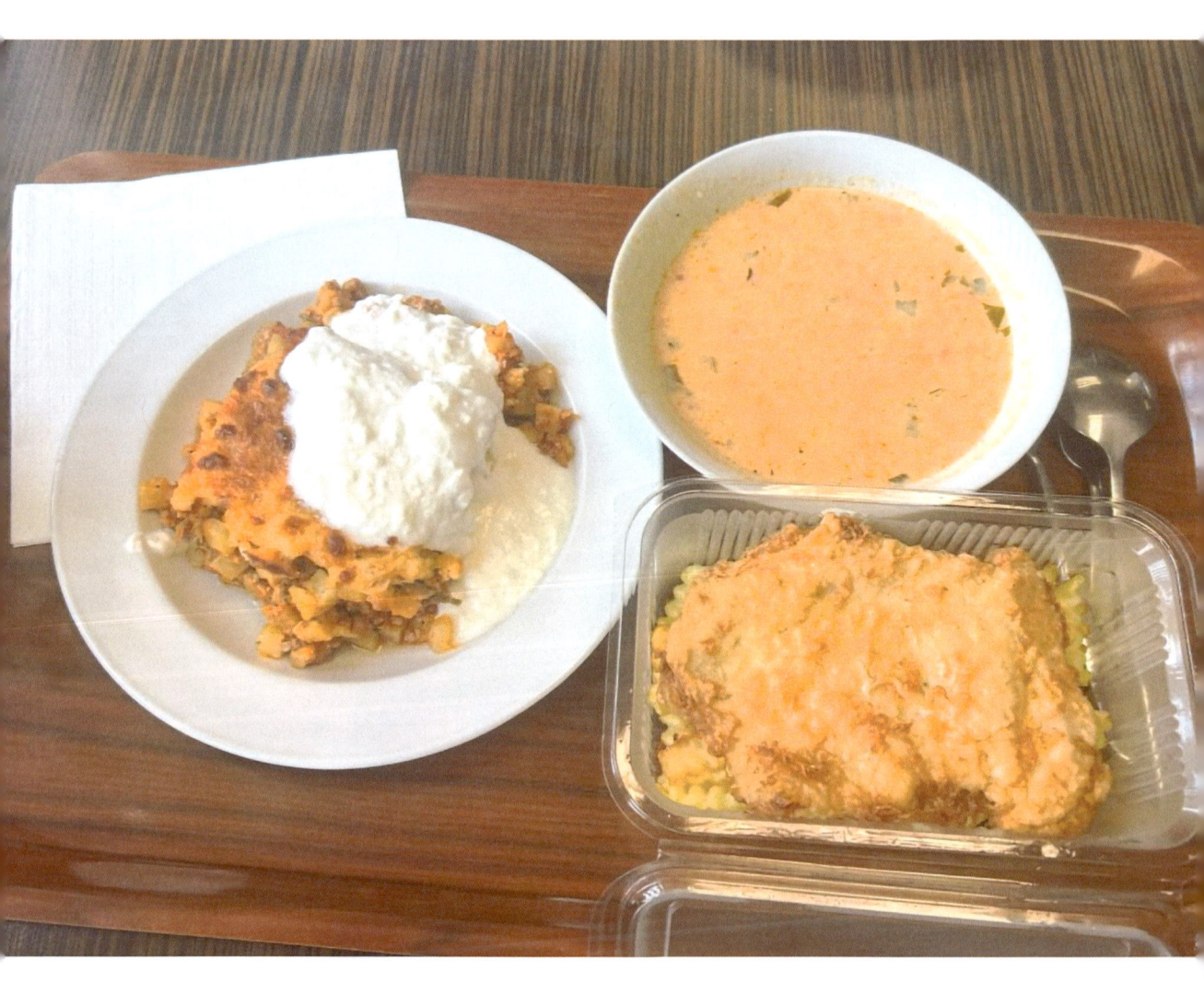

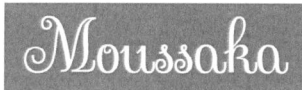

Moussaka

INGREDIENTS

Two pounds ground beef or lamb, four yellow potatoes, one onion, celery, one carrot, one red pepper, one tomato, 5 cloves of garlic, salt, black pepper, turmeric, cardamon, coriander, savory or oregano, sweet paprika, tomato sauce, vegetable broth, parsley, one cup yogurt, two eggs, two soup spoons flour, olive oil.

Boil the potatoes for 15 min. on medium, peel and cut into cubes.

Chop the onion, celery, carrot, red pepper, tomato and garlic. Add salt and black pepper. Mix and sauté in a pan with covered lid in heated olive oil for 10 min. on medium. Add the ground meat, and the remaining spices, mix and cook for another 10 min.

Layer the potatoes in a baking dish sprayed with olive oil, then the vegetable mixture, then potatoes again. Pour ½ can of tomato sauce on top or a layer with sliced tomatoes. Evenly pour vegetable broth to cover the lower layer of potatoes.

In a mixer, mix the eggs well with the yogurt, flour and salt. Pour evenly over the layers of potatoes and meat mixture. Bake until the top has a golden color. Serve with yogurt or sour cream. Sprinkle with chopped parsley.

Schnitzel is described on another page.

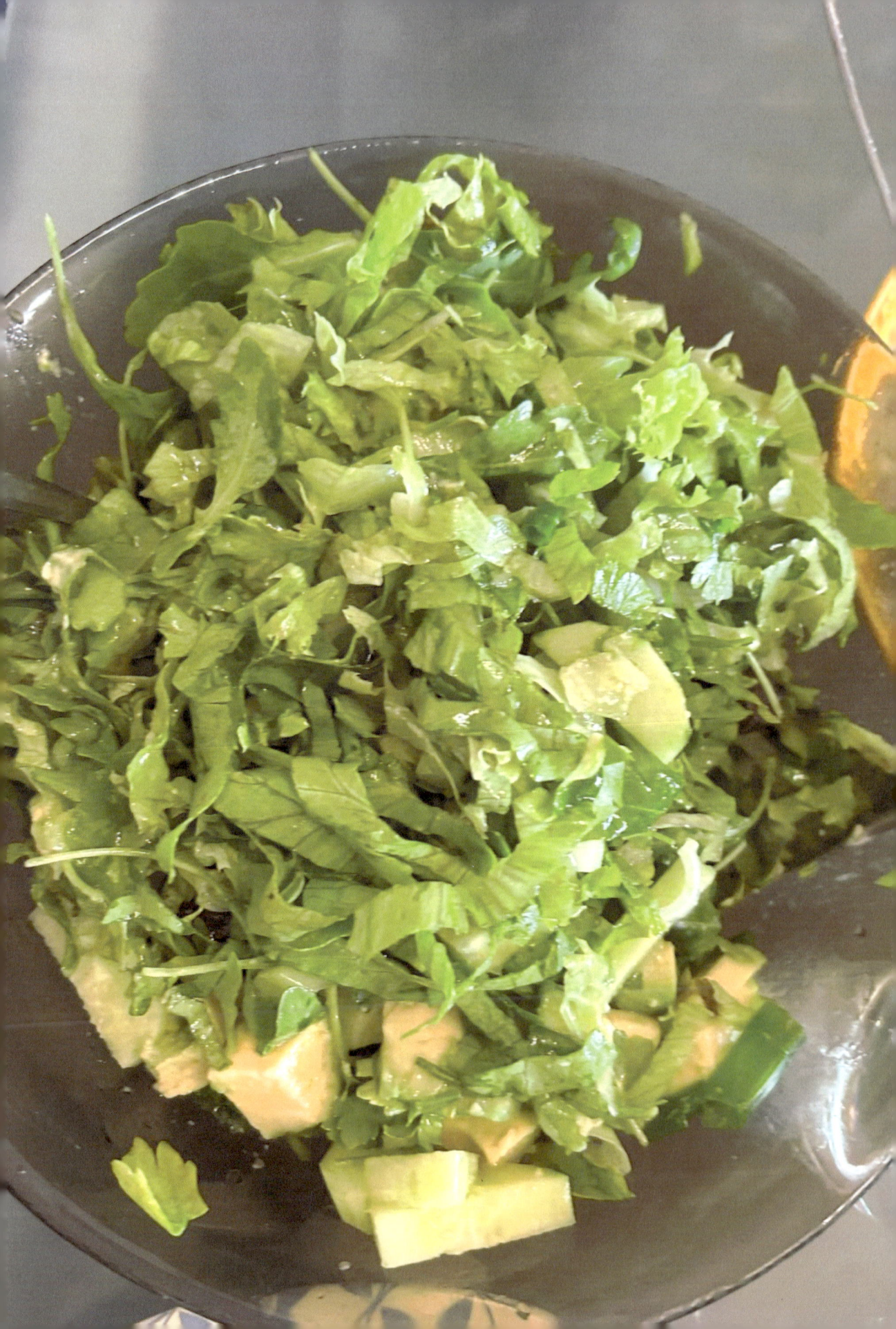

Green Salad With Avocado and Cucumbers

INGREDIENTS

Chopped green salad, peeled and sliced cucumbers in small cubes, sliced avocado, dressing: 1 teaspoon olive oil, teaspoon of vinegar. or squeezed lemon, salt.

Mix all ingredients in a bowl, prepare the dressing in a separate bowl and pour over the salad. The salad is easy to prepare and a healthy and beautiful addition to a main dish of meat.

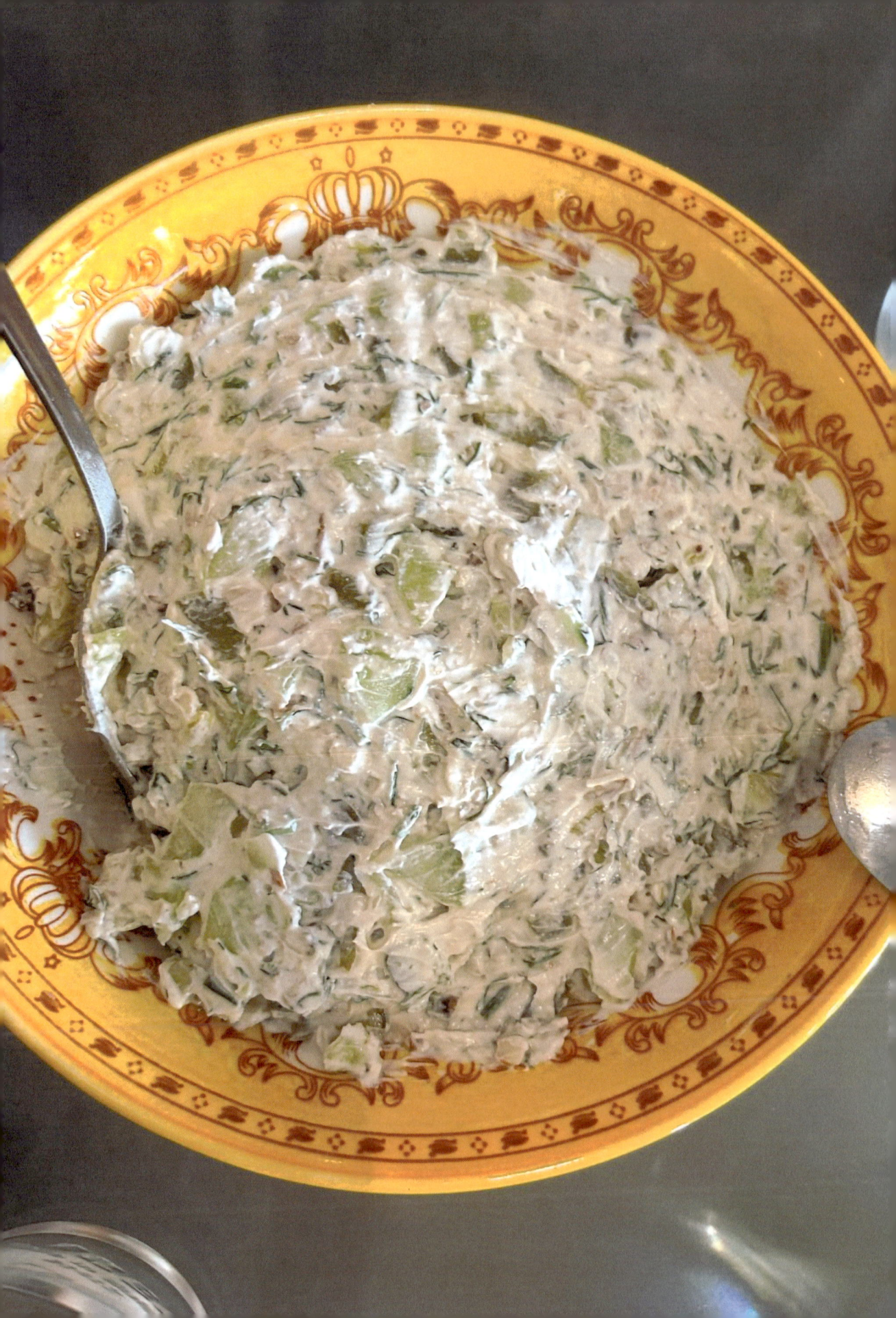

Chicken with Sour Cream and Pickles

INGREDIENTS

One-pound boiled chicken breast, one cup of sour cream, three pickles, olive oil, dill.

Cut the chicken breast into cubes or small slices, mix with sour cream, cut pickles into small cubes, add dill. You may also add cooked peas and carrots cut into small cubes. Serve with baked potatoes.

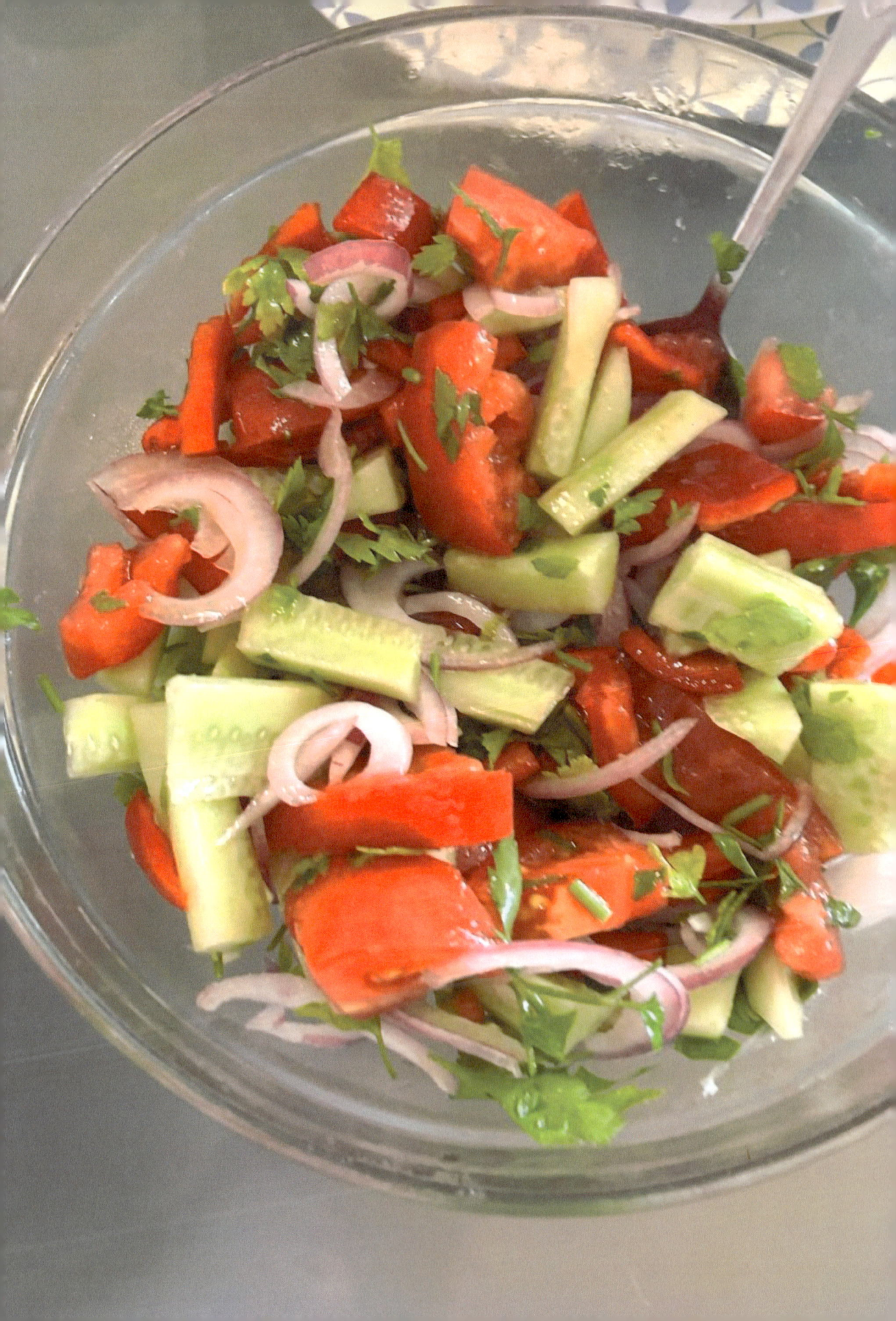

Tomato And Cucumber Salad

INGREDIENTS

Chopped tomatoes, peeled and cut cucumber, red onion cut in thin slices, parsley, vinaigrette dressing of olive oil, vinegar, and a pinch of salt

Mix all ingredients, pour the vinaigrette dressing on top, garnish with parsley.

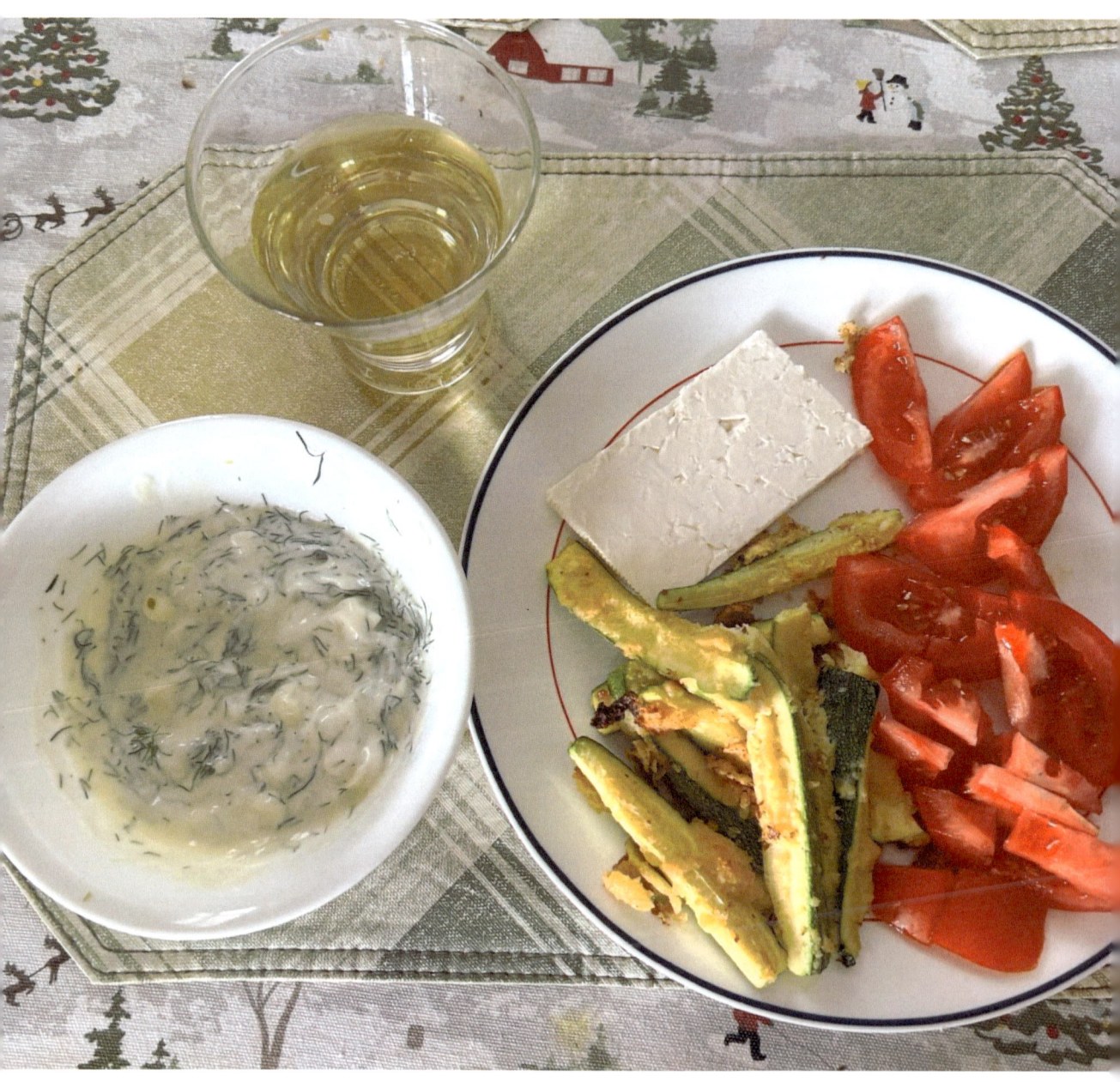

Baked Zucchini, Feta Cheese, Tomatoes, Dill Sauce

INGREDIENTS

Washed zucchini sliced vertically, two cut tomatoes, a block of feta cheese, two eggs, flour, breadcrumbs, olive oil, a cup of yogurt, tablespoon of mayo, finely chopped garlic, dill.

Dip the zucchini slices one by one in the flour, shake off the flour, then dip in whisked eggs, and then the breadcrumbs, place on a baking flat dish sprayed with olive oil, bake and broil at 390 degrees until golden in color.

Mix the yogurt, mayo, garlic, and dill well.

Arrange the food on a serving dish and serve with chilled white wine, yogurt drink or apple juice.

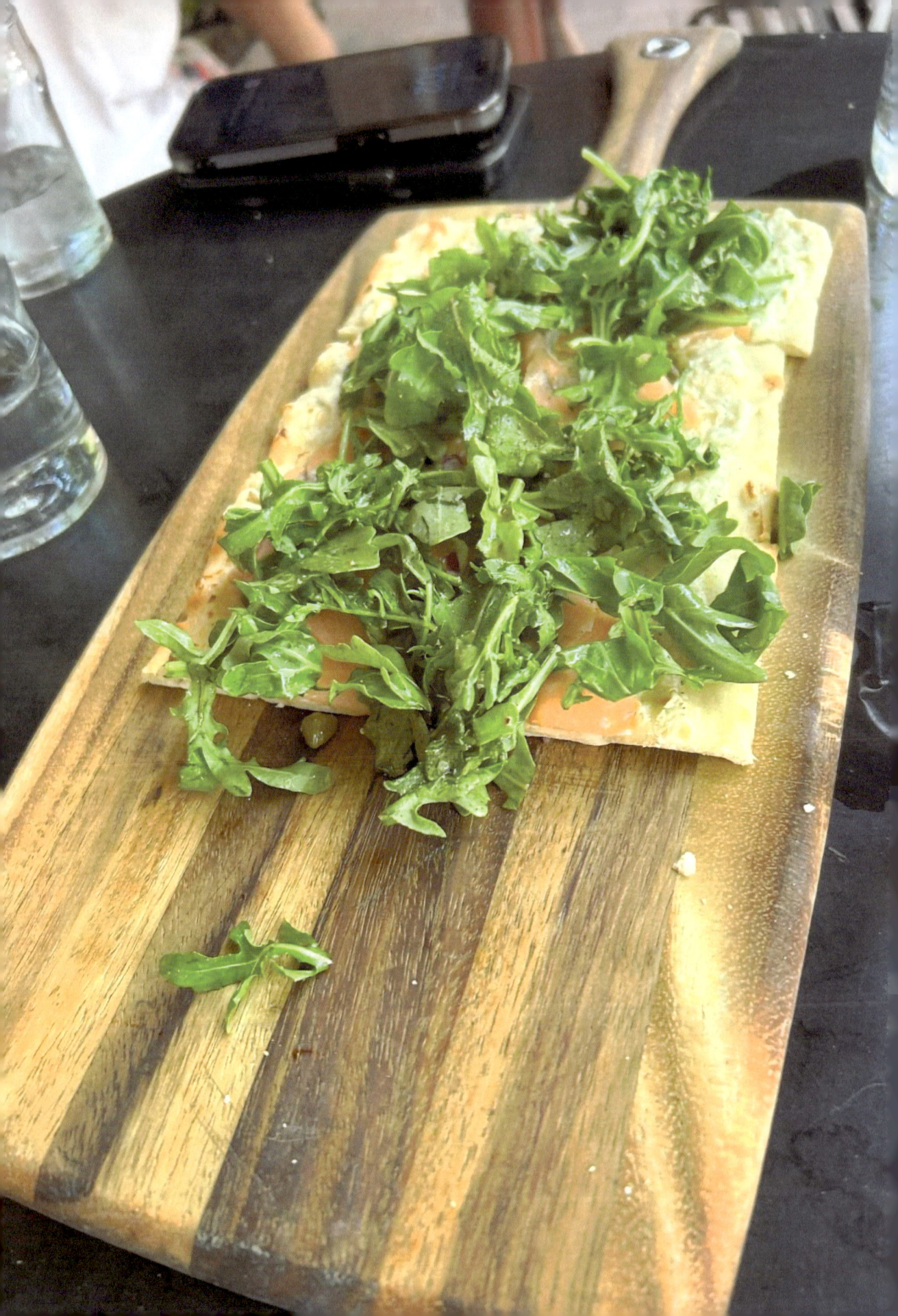

Smoked Salmon On Pita Bread

INGREDIENTS

Smoked salmon, flat pita bread, hummus, chopped lettuce.

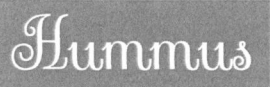

INGREDIENTS

Chickpeas cooked or from a can, one squeezed lemon, ¼ cup tahini – ground sesame seeds, oil, salt mixed in a food processor, then add ½ teaspoon cumin, sweet paprika, sumac, two tablespoons of cold water, mix well.

Spread hummus on the pita bread, follow with smoked salmon, and top with lettuce,

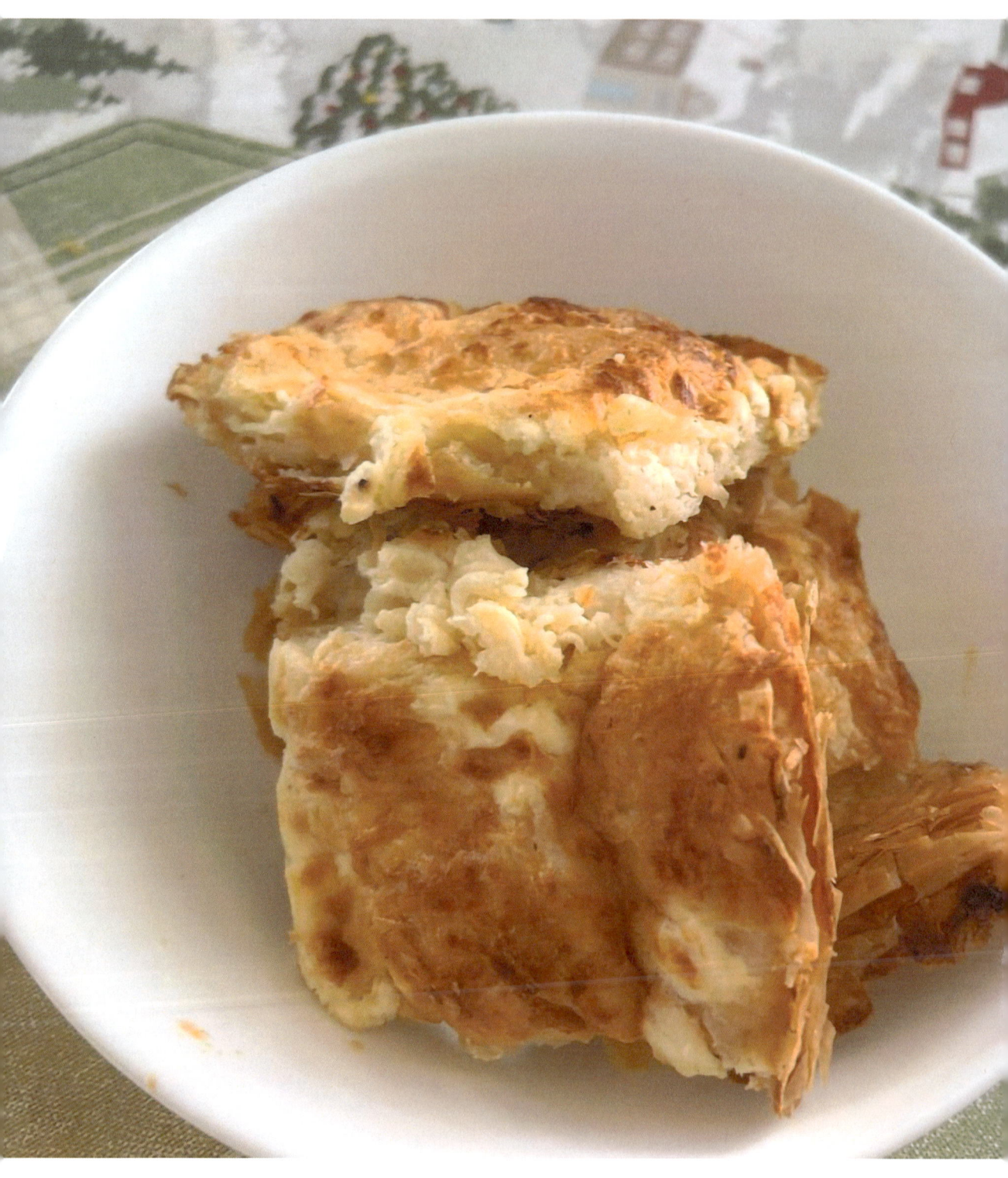

Milk Banitsa

—————————————————————

Phyllo dough, (a package from store of home prepared) two cups of milk, two eggs, one cup sugar, vanilla extract, half a stick of butter, one tablespoon powdered sugar.

Melt the butter and cover the baking pan lightly with the melted butter. Layer two sheets of the dough and brush with butter, continue until all sheets are used up. Cut into rectangular or square forms and bake at 370 degrees until the top has a golden color.

Mix the eggs with the sugar in a mixer, then add slightly warmed milk, and the vanilla extract, mix until the sugar is absorbed. Pour over the baked layers of dough and bake 10-15 min at 340 degrees. Take out of the oven and sprinkle with powdered sugar.

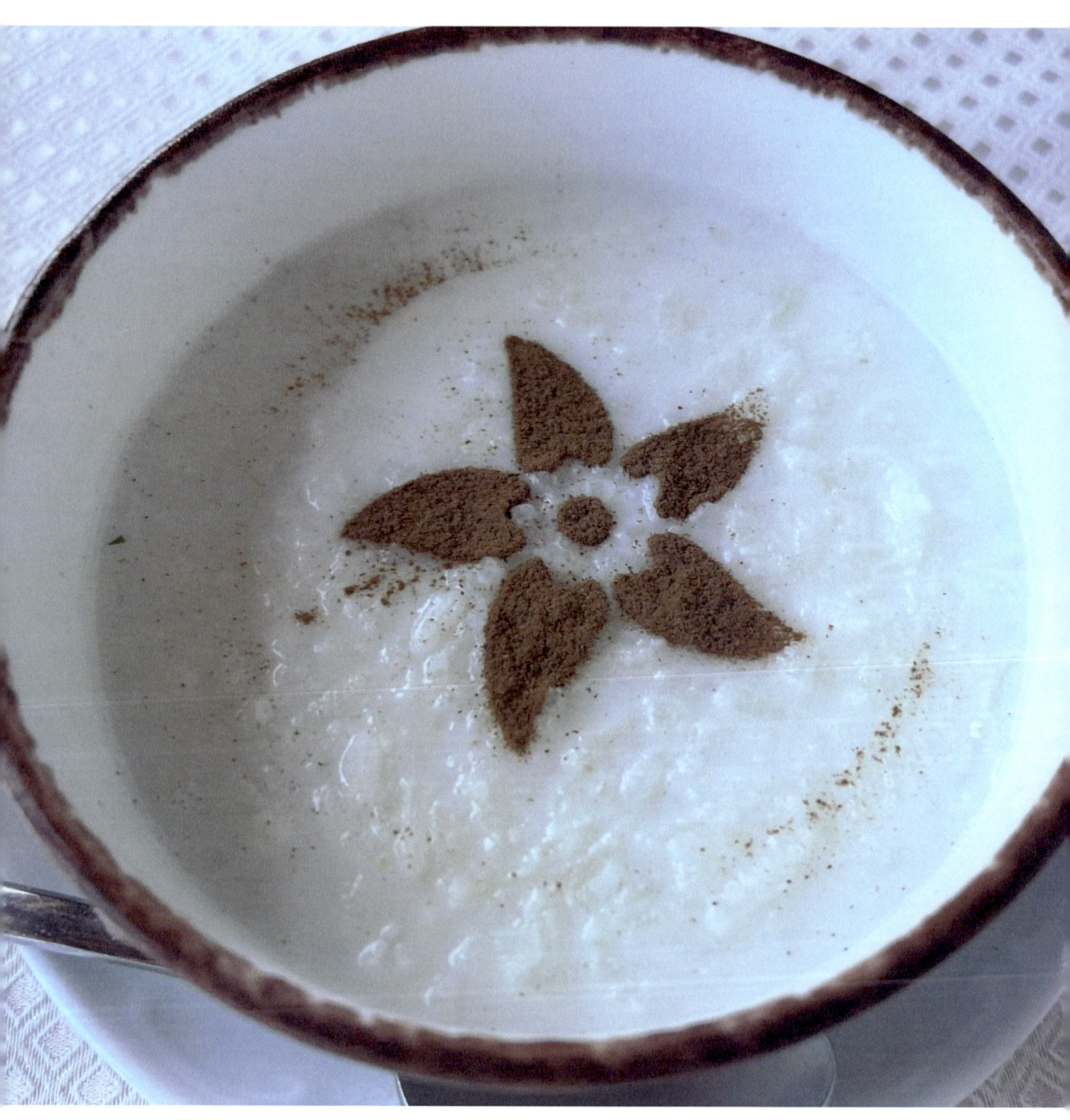

Sutliash or Rice and Milk Dessert

INGREDIENTS

500 ml water, 600 ml milk, 200 g white rice, vanilla extract, cinnamon, two teaspoons sugar, a pinch of salt.

Boil the rice with salt and water until the water evaporates, pour in the milk, the vanilla extract, and the sugar and cook until rice thickens, decorate with cinnamon.

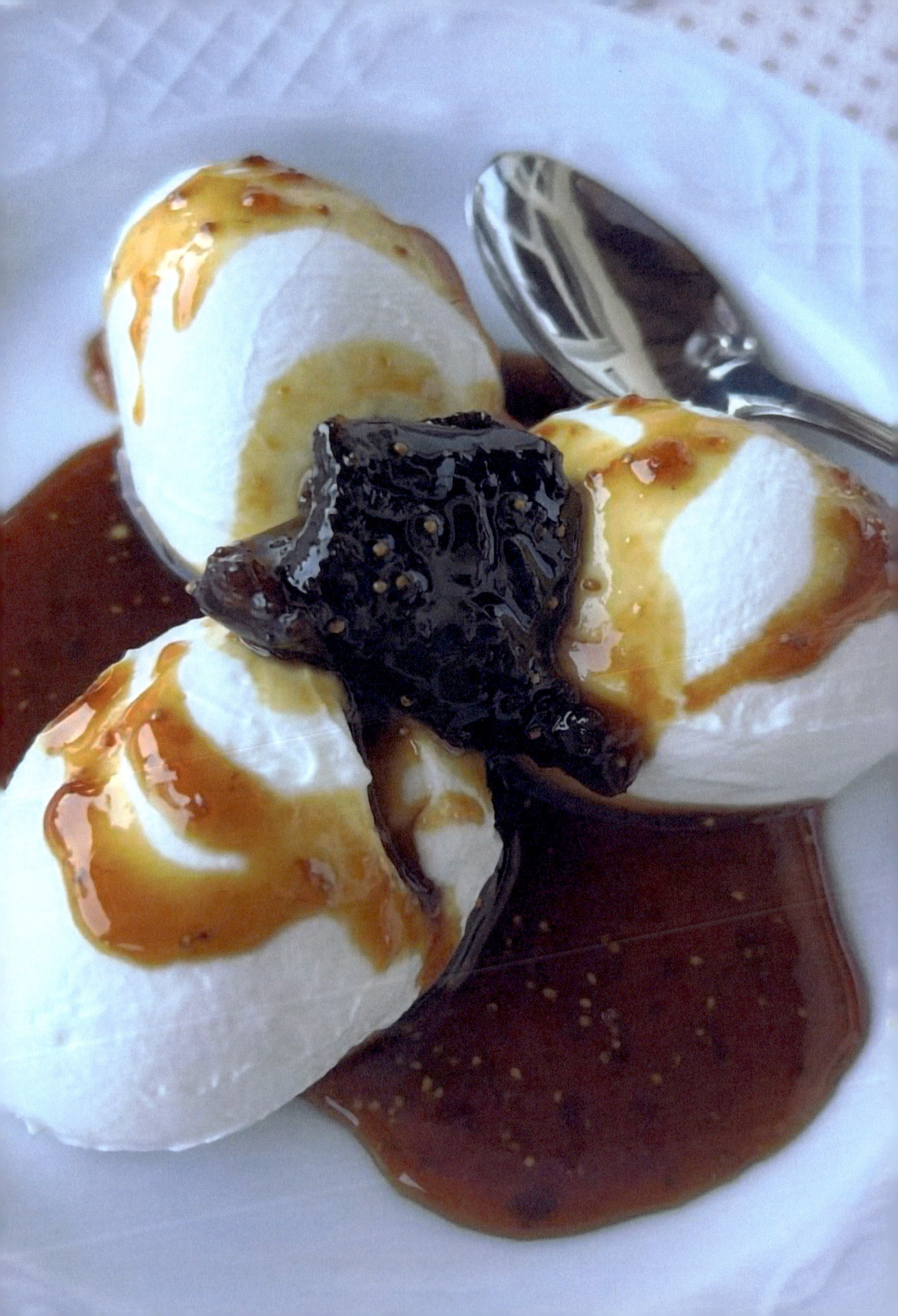

Scoops of Frozen Yogurt with Raspberry Jam and Fig Preserves

INGREDIENTS AND SERVING

Frozen yogurt from the store, or prepared by mixing whole milk yogurt with mascarpone, cup of sugar, vanilla extract, teaspoon of corn syrup, freeze in a container. When frozen, scoop and serve on a bed of raspberry jam, spray with fig jam and add fig preserves in the middle.

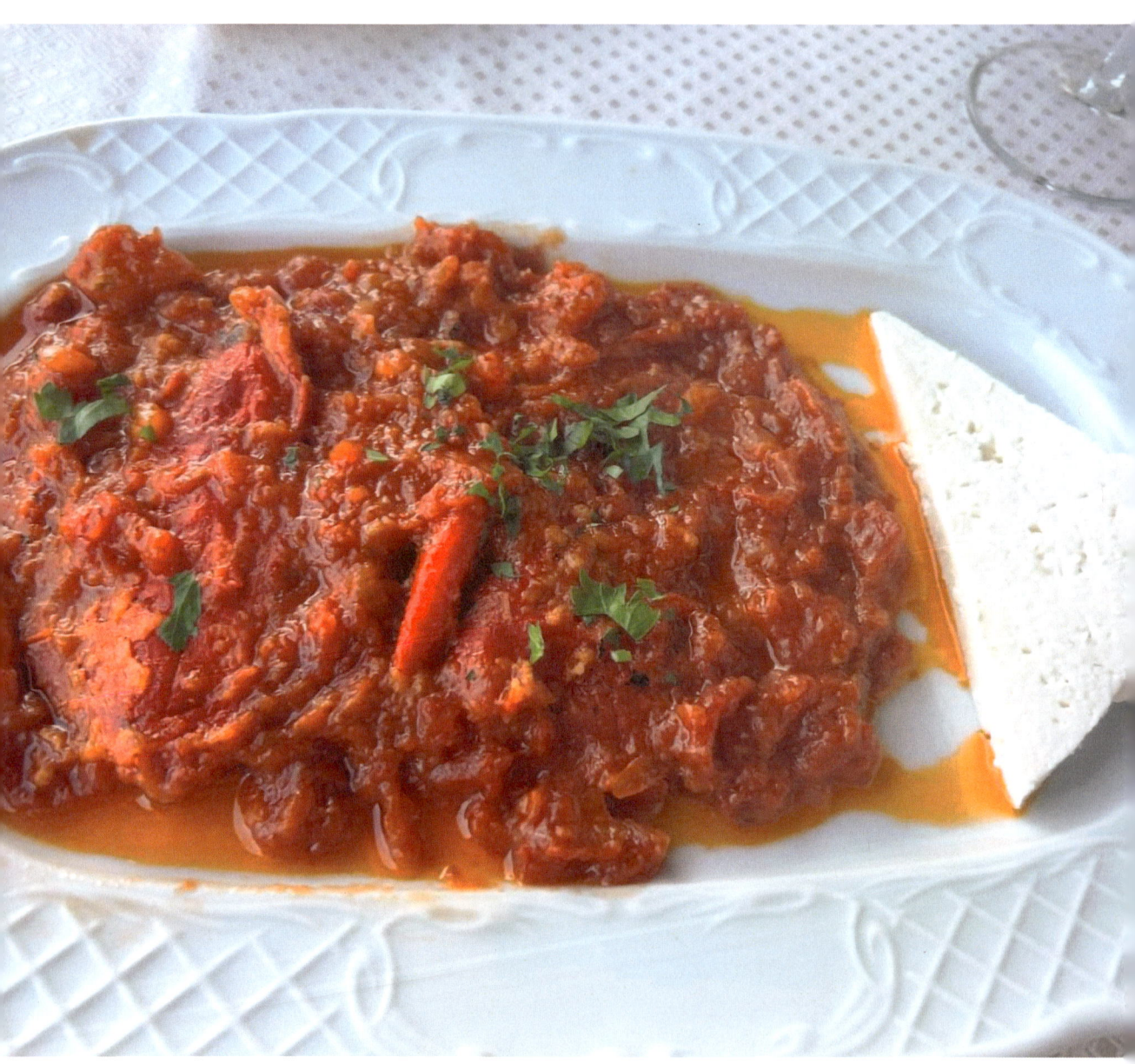

Mish Mash with Block of Feta Cheese

INGREDIENTS

Four tomatoes, four red peppers, one eggplant, four eggs, one onion, one tablespoon olive oil, salt.

Peel and cut the eggplant in cubes, salt and let rest, dice and simmer the onion on the stove in a pan with heated oil on low heat for five minutes. Add the eggplant, the sliced peppers and diced tomatoes. Cook until the water evaporates, crack and add the eggs, stir and cook for another five min. or less as you prefer the consistency of the eggs. Garnish with parsley, add a block of feta cheese on the side.

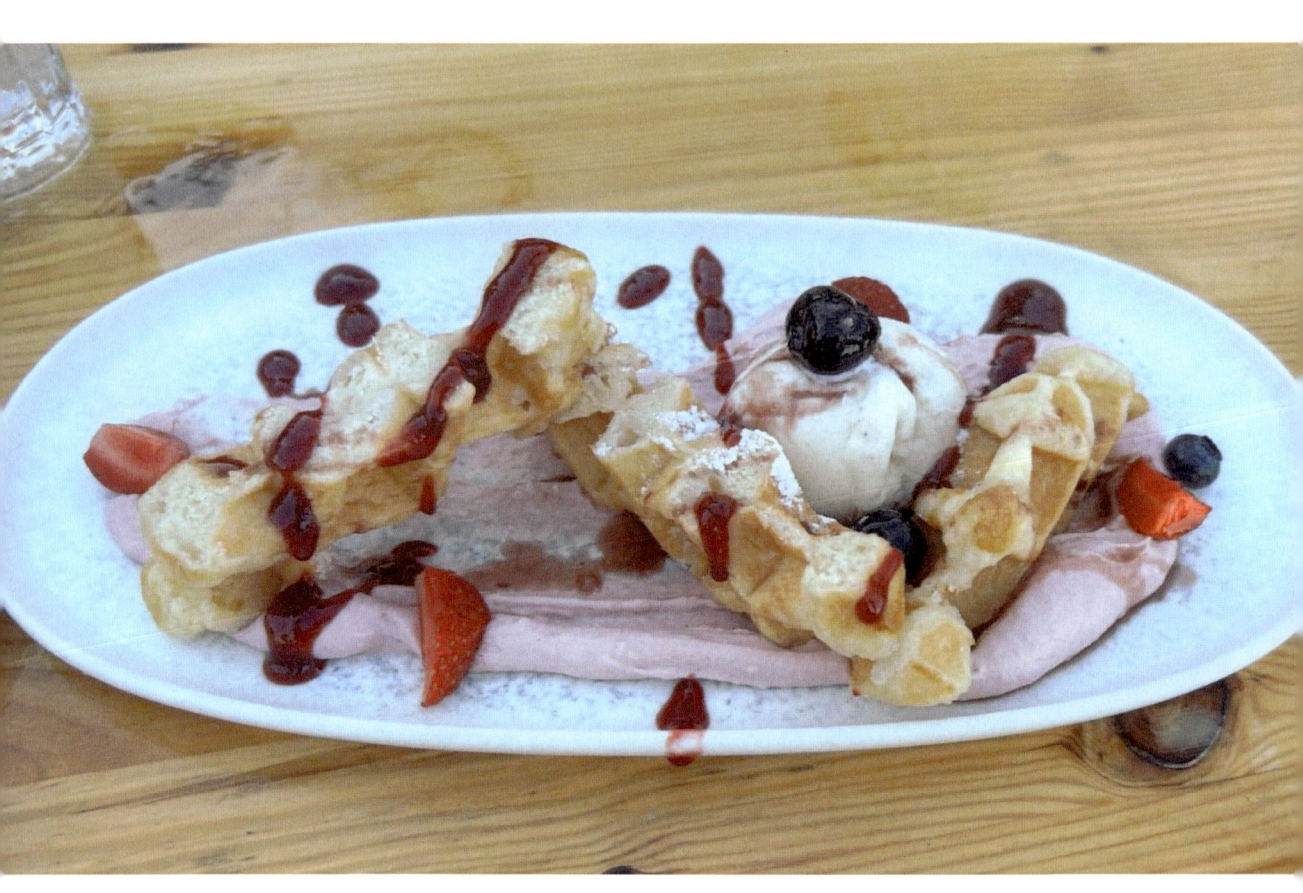

Waffle Sticks with Frozen Ice Cream and Berries

INGREDIENTS

Waffle sticks bought or prepared. Prepare in waffle maker: one egg, milk, vanilla, cinnamon, brioche bread. Spray the waffle maker with oil and preheat, in a bowl beat the egg, whisk in the milk, sugar, vanilla and cinnamon, dip the slice of bread into the mixture and place in waffle maker, cook 3-4 min. until golden brown. Repeat with the rest of the slices.

Mix a scoop of frozen vanilla yogurt and raspberry jam and spread on the bottom of the serving dish. Place a couple of scoops of frozen yogurt on top, decorate with waffle sticks and berries – blueberry and raspberry.

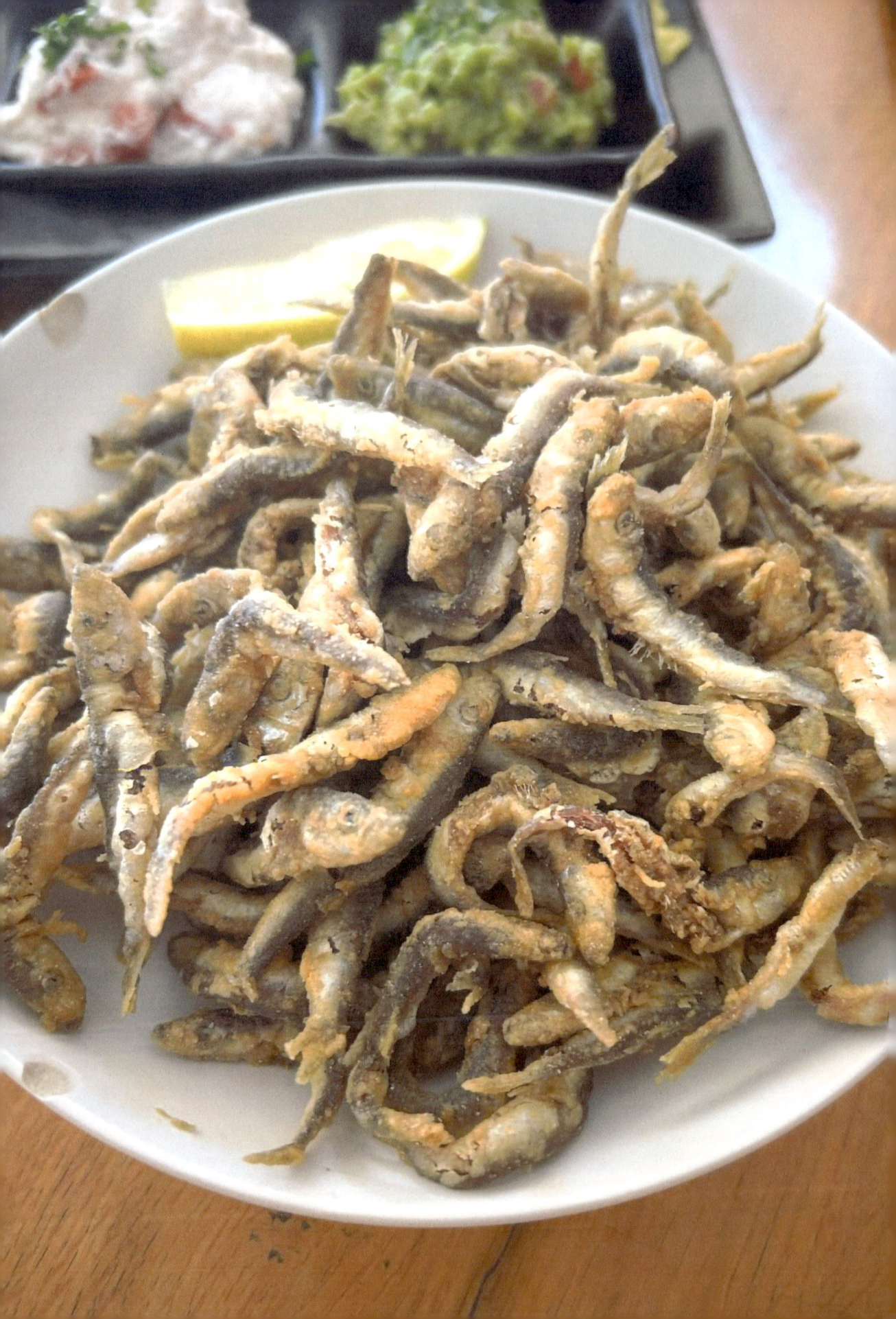

Black Sea Sprat
(Sardines, Atlantic Herring)

INGREDIENTS

One kilo fish, 2-3 tablespoons of flour, two tablespoons of corn flour, salt, garlic powder, oil, bay leaf.

Roll the clean fish in the mixture of flour, corn flour, salt and garlic powder. Heat the oil on the stove, place in a couple of bay leaves, and place the fish in the heated oil one by one, cook until golden brown, serve with slices of lemon and green salad.

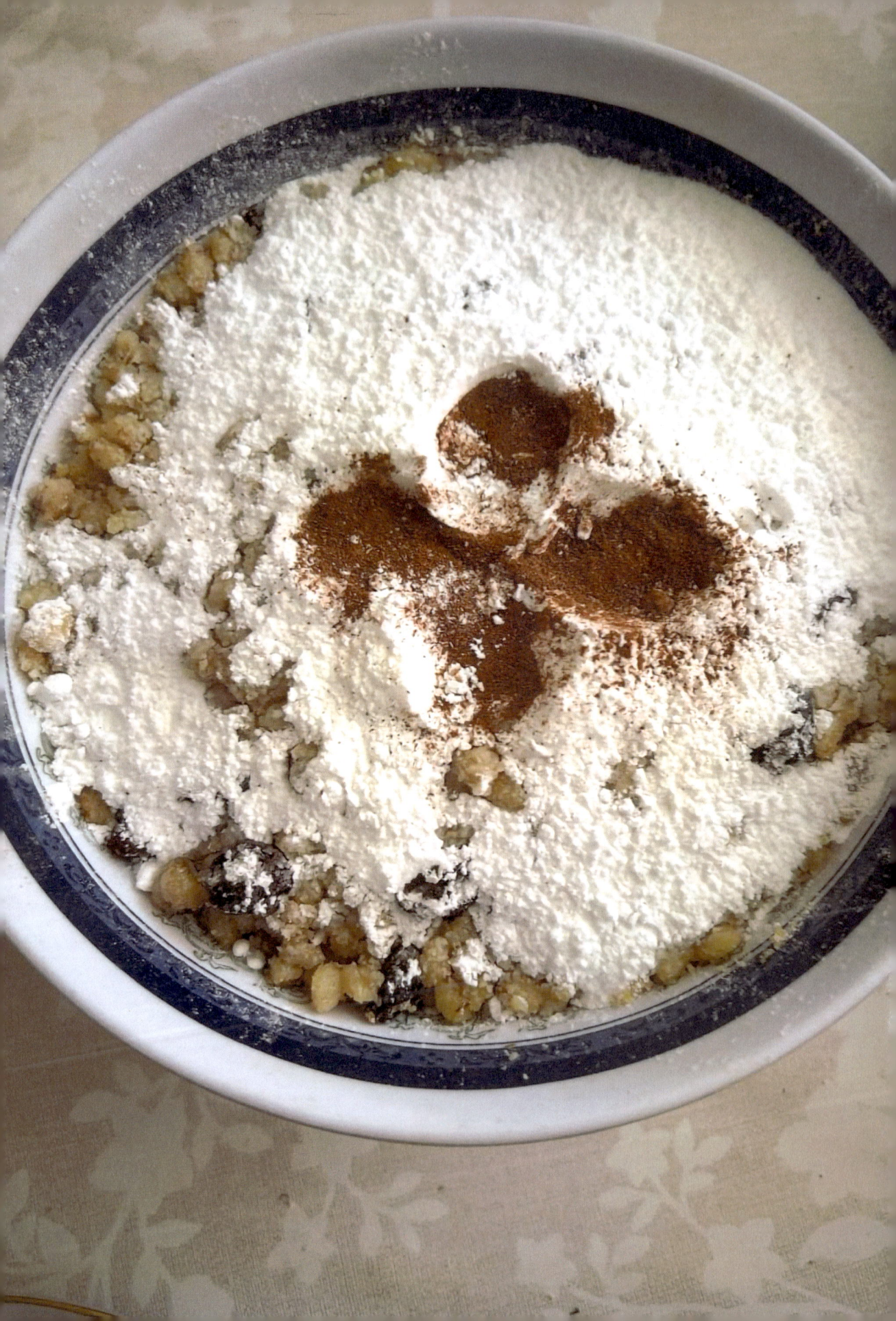

Boiled Wheat with Cinnamon

INGREDIENTS ────────────────────────────

Wheat or barley 50 g, one tablespoon sugar, salt, raisins, walnuts, vanilla extract, grated lemon peel, powdered sugar, cinnamon.

Boil the wheat in water with a pinch of salt until the grains crack, drain the water and add the sugar, minced walnuts, grated lemon peel and mix well. spread powder sugar on top and make a cross with the cinnamon. This dish is used on Eastern Orthodox religious holidays to commemorate the dead.

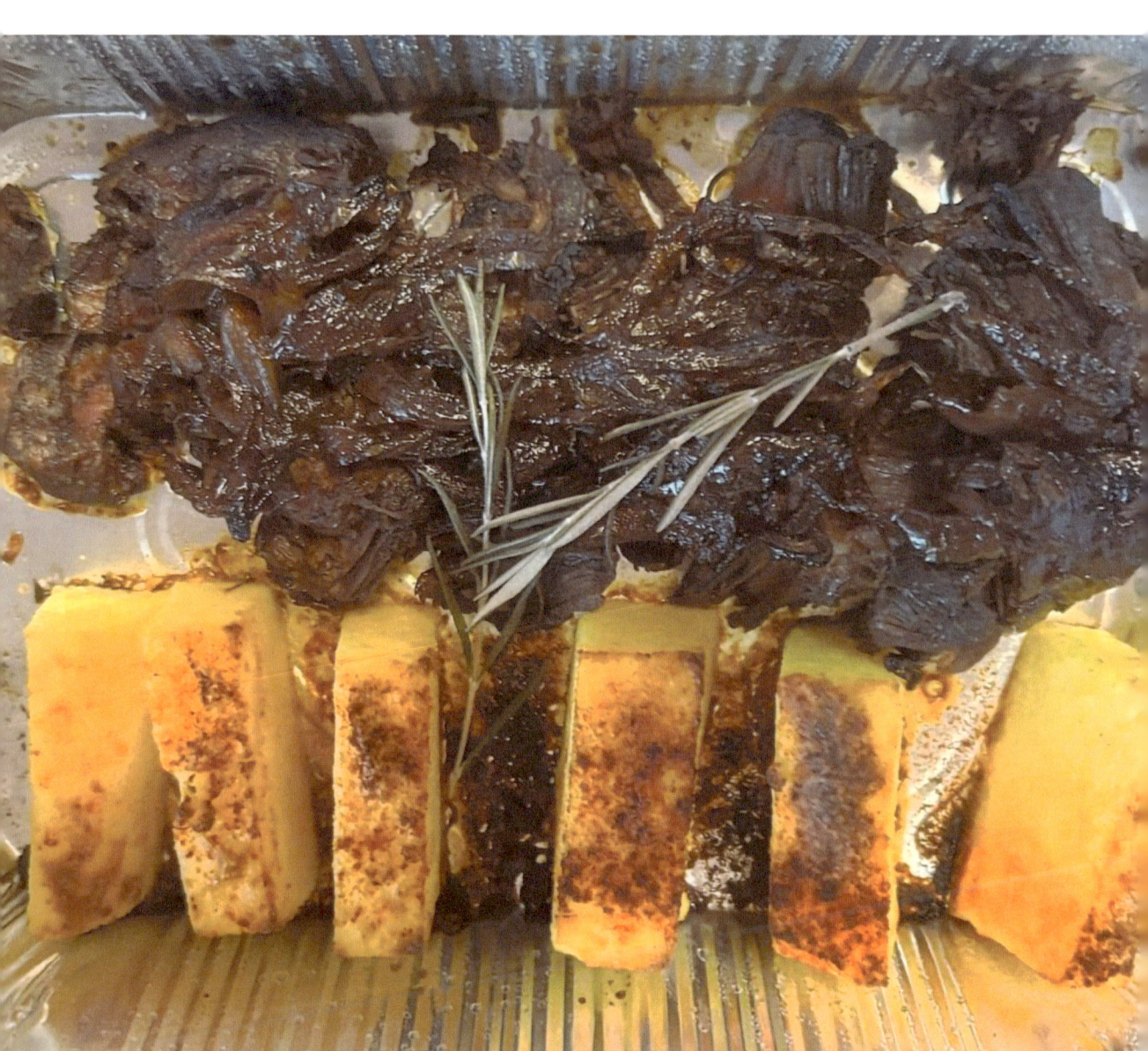

Baked Rack of Ribs with Polenta

INGREDIENTS

Pork ribs 1 kg, soy sauce 1 tablespoon, mustard, ketchup 1 tablespoon, honey 1 teaspoon, garlic powder, cumin, black pepper, sweet paprika, a little water.

Mix all the spices and rub on the ribs. Cover with foil and refrigerate for an hour. Bake at 400 degrees until browned, turn over to bake on both sides.

Polenta recipe is on another page

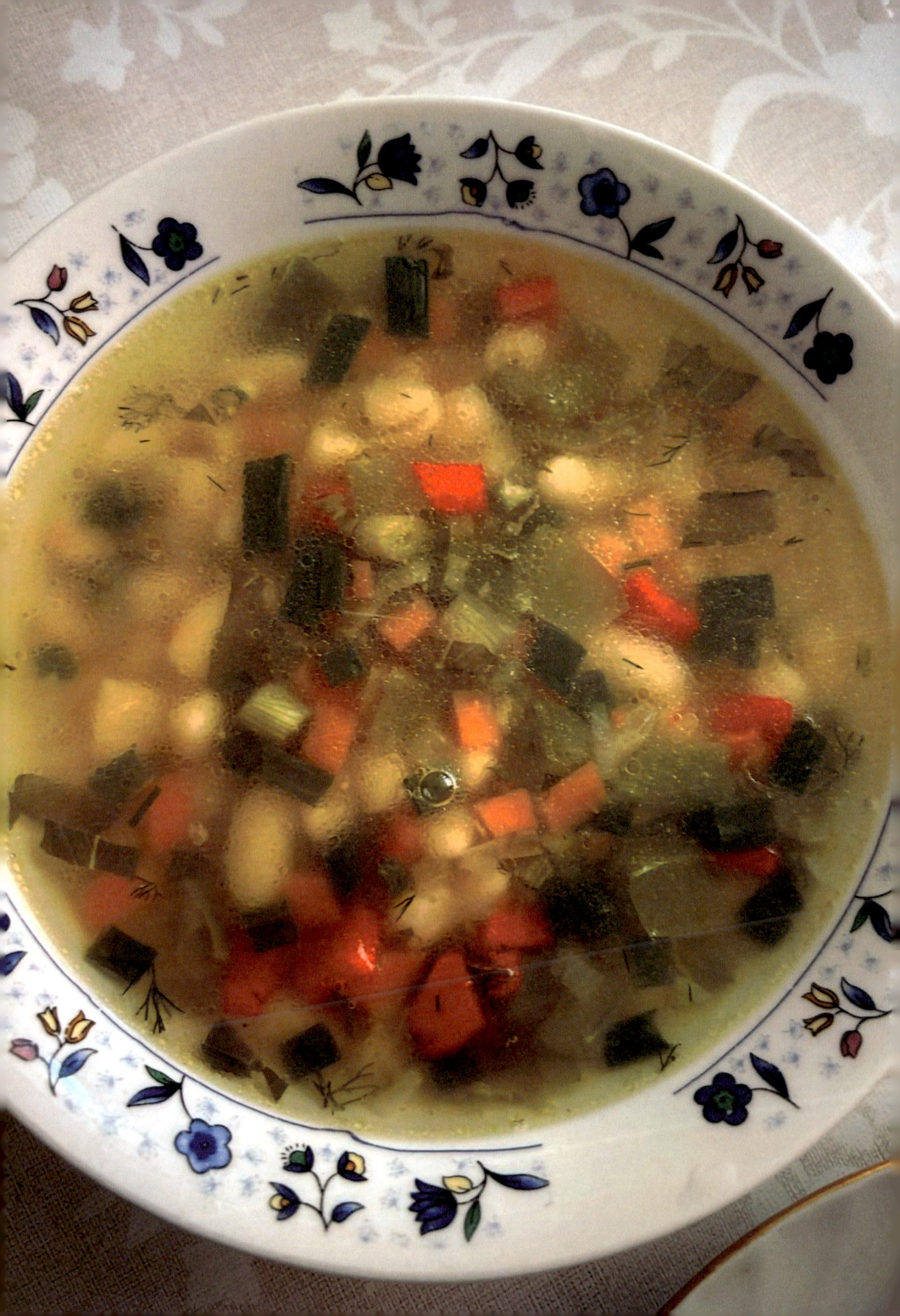

Vegetable Soup with Beans

INGREDIENTS AND PREPARATION

Dice red and green peppers, celery, two fresh onions and two carrots, add salt and black pepper and simmer in a pot greased with olive oil for 5 minutes, add one cup of white beans, parsley, chicken or vegetable broth to cover the mixture. Boil 15-20 min. on medium heat. Garnish with parsley.

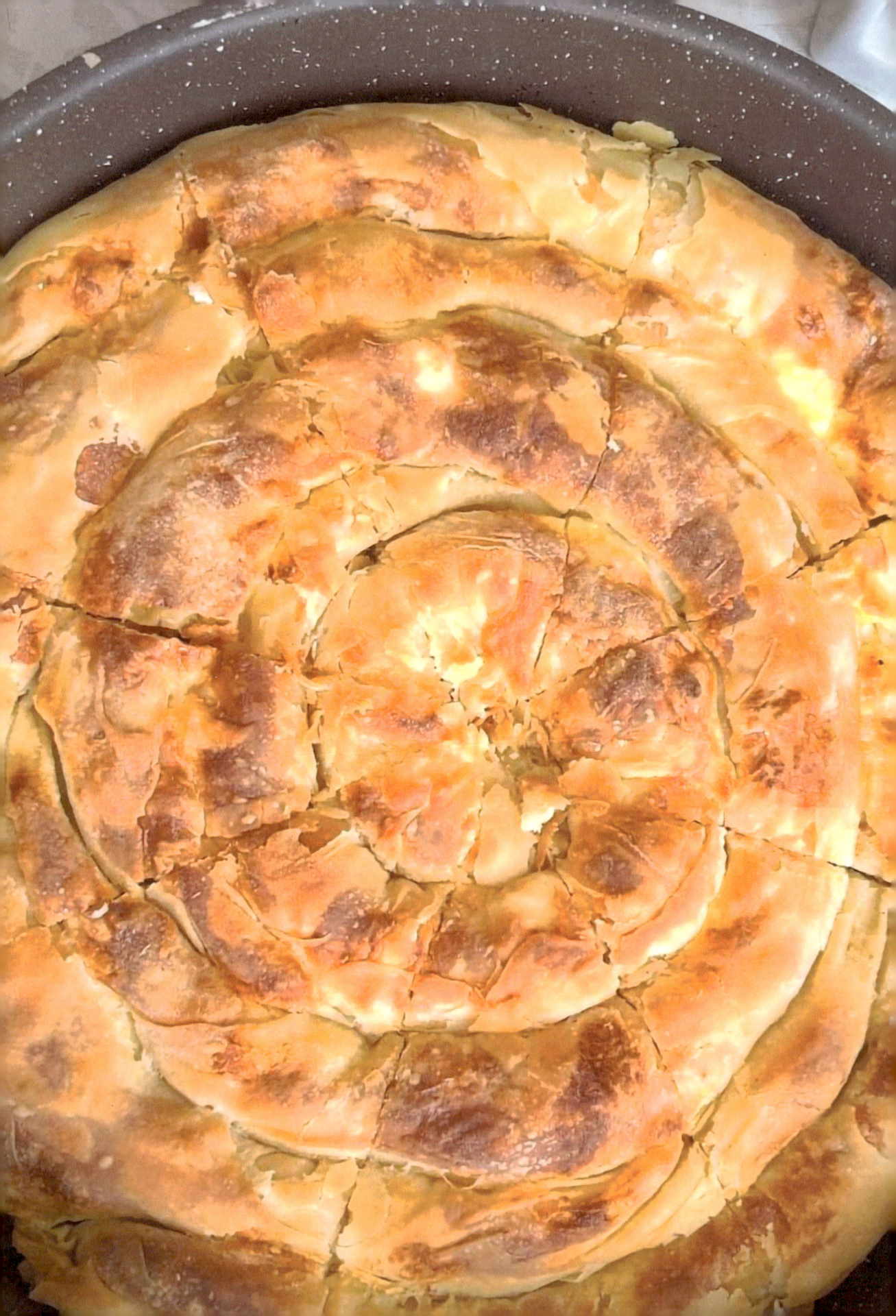

Banitsa - Phyllo Dough Filled with Feta Cheese, Yogurt and Eggs, Favorite Bulgarian and Balkan Dish

Dish Found At Bakeries All Over The Cities In Bulgaria

INGREDIENTS

Phyllo dough is available in the frozen section of most supermarkets, or it can be prepared from scratch. Half a stick melted butter, 3 eggs, 5 tablespoons yogurt, 300 g crumbled feta cheese, ½ teaspoon baking soda. (You may add a couple of tablespoons of ricotta or cottage cheese)

Mix all the ingredients well in a bowl.

Open the dough on a flat surface, take the edge of three sheets from one corner, overlap on top so that when you roll the dough it will always be three sheets at the time.

Spread the cheese mixture vertically with a spoon in the middle of the top sheet and roll the three sheets to form a funnel like shape. Arrange in a circle in a greased pan with olive oil. Continue until all sheets are used.

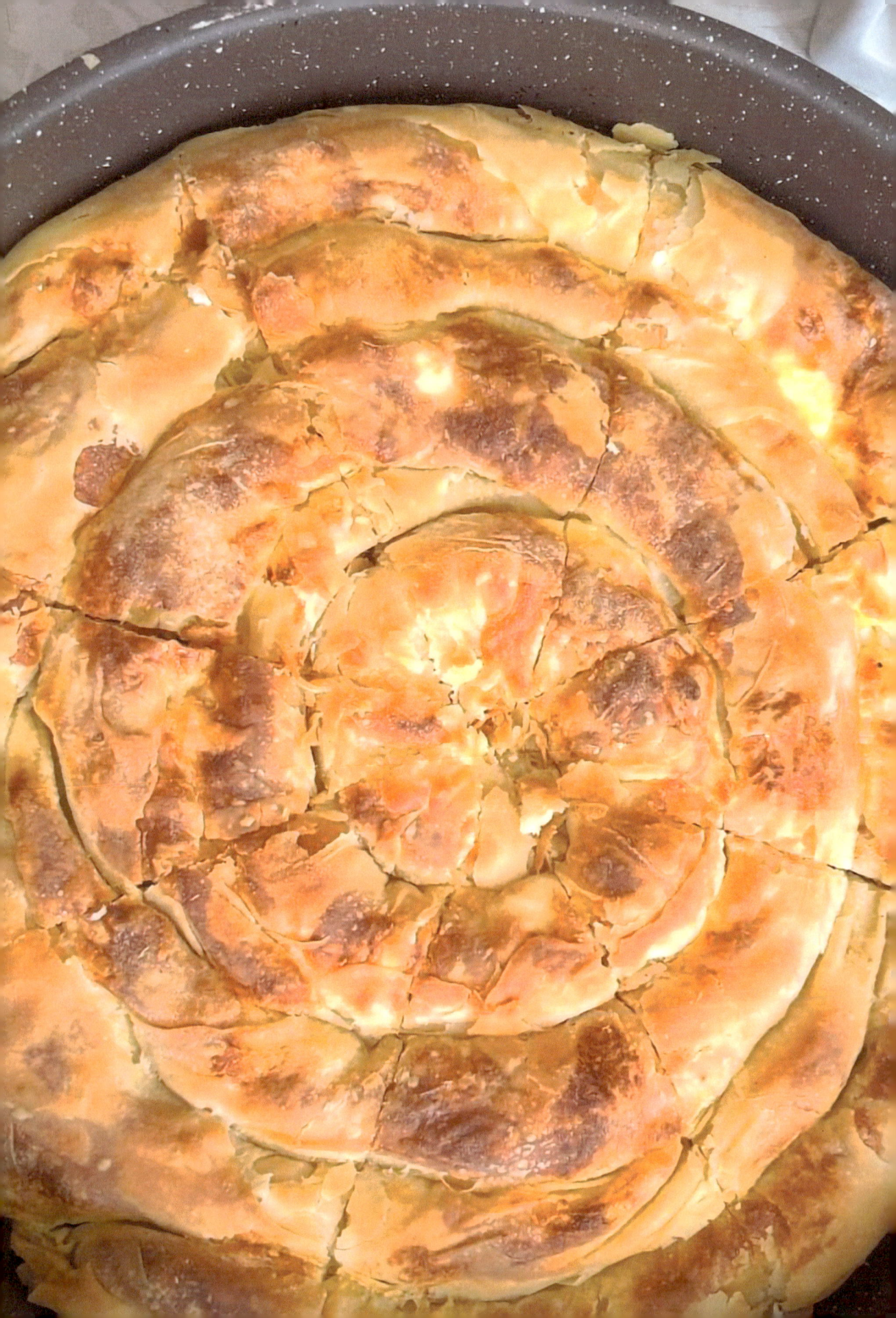

Mix one egg with three tablespoons of yogurt and spread evenly on the top. Bake at 370 degrees for 20 minutes, reduce to 330 degrees for another 10 min. or until the banitsa has a golden reddish color.

Serve with a yogurt drink.

Ingredients for Homemade Dough:

400 g flour, one
egg, ½ teaspoon vinegar, 50 ml water, oil

In a bowl, add the flour, the egg, the vinegar, and a little water to prepare the dough. Leave the dough greased on top for half an hour at room temperature. Then break it into balls, grease a flat clean surface on the table and roll each ball until it becomes a thin sheet. Continue with the rest of the dough balls.

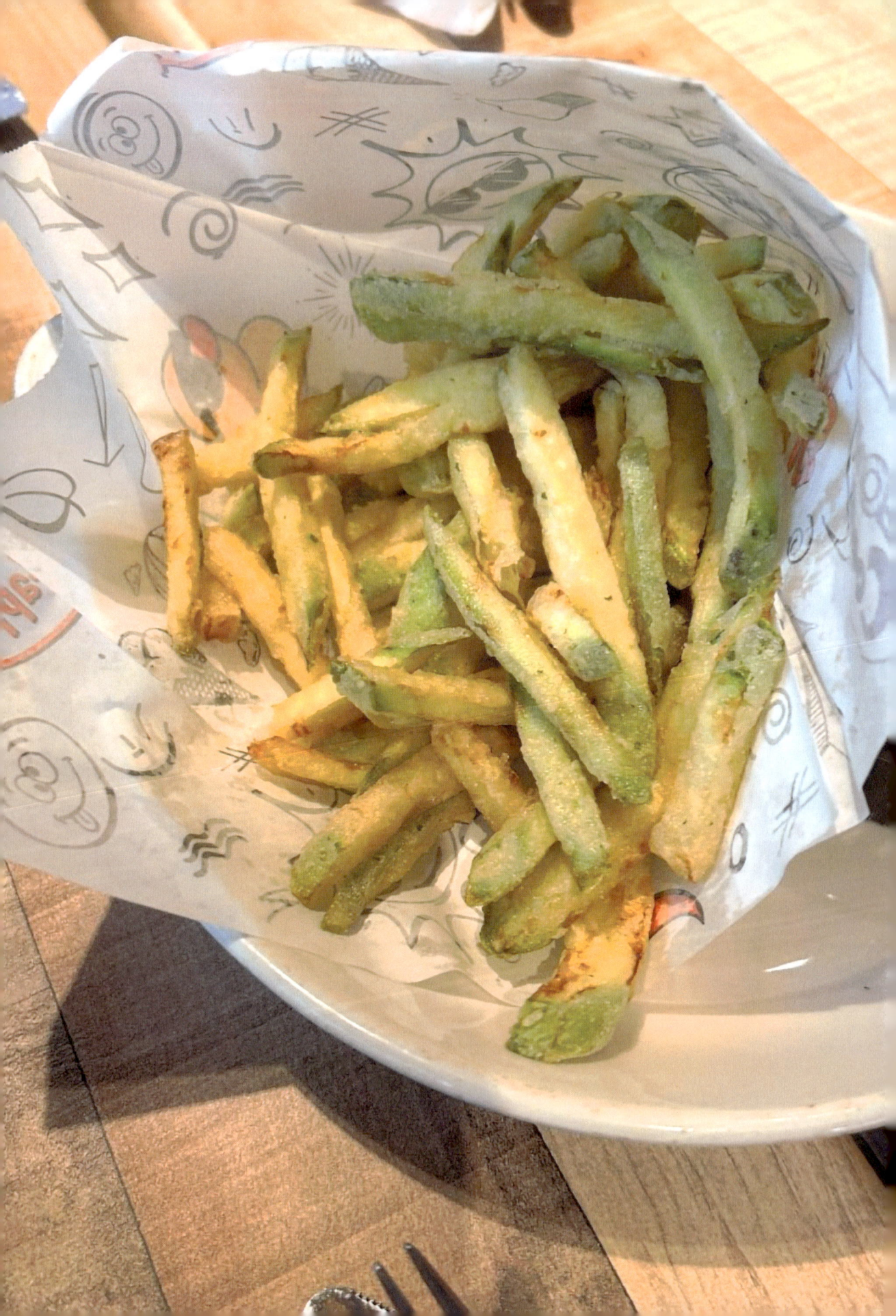

Zucchini Sticks

INGREDIENTS

Two zucchinis, two tablespoons corn flour, one tablespoon flour, two eggs, salt.

Mix all the ingredients for the mixture and dip the vertically sliced zucchini in it one by one. Place on a baking sheet and bake at 390 degrees until golden brown. Serve with mayo, yogurt and dill dip.

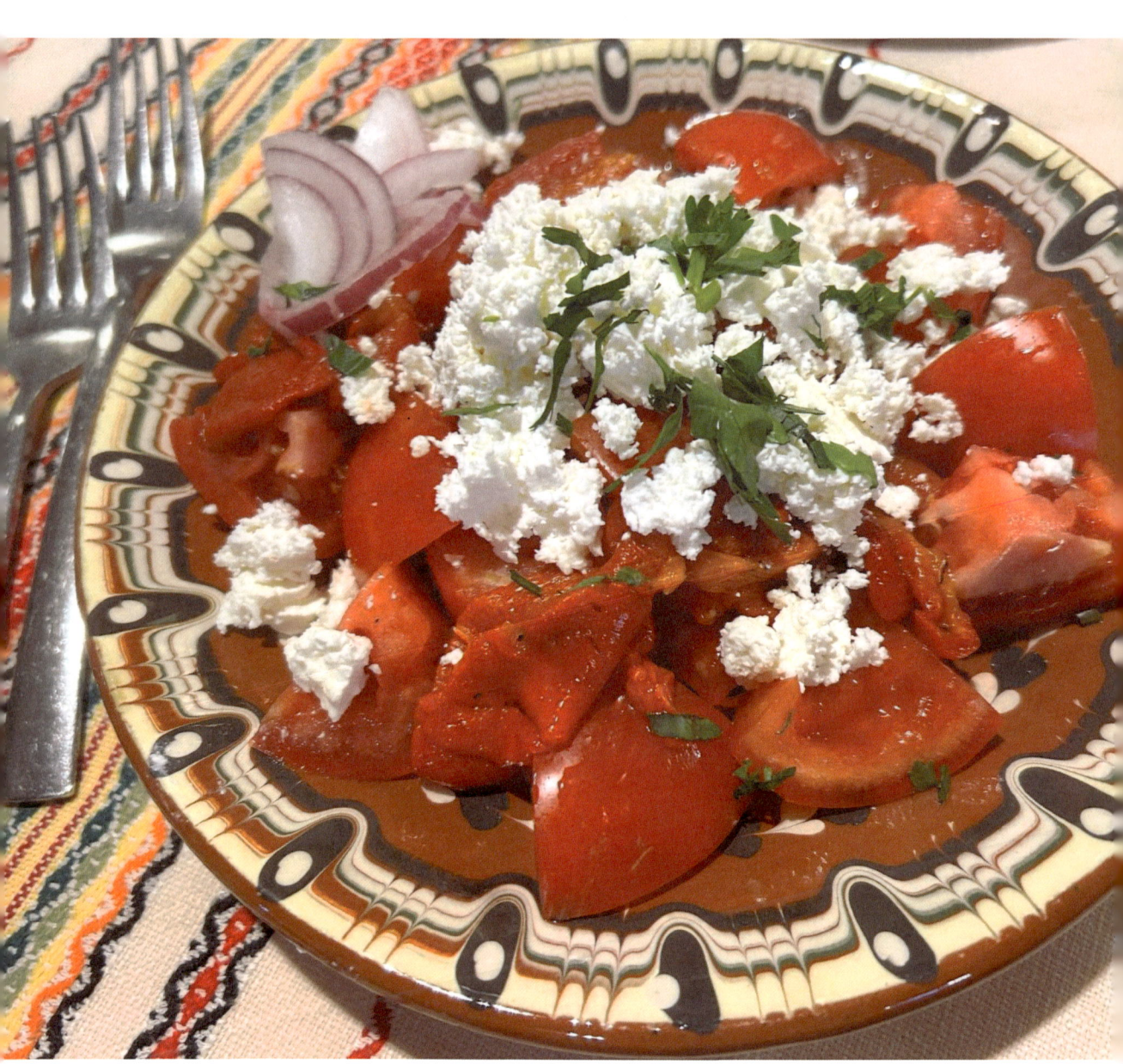

Tomatoes and Pepper Salad

INGREDIENTS

Sliced tomatoes, baked, peeled and sliced red peppers, crumbled feta cheese, sliced red onion, parsley, vinaigrette dressing – vinegar or lemon juice, olive oil, pinch of salt.

Arrange the cut tomatoes and peppers in a serving dish. Evenly pour the vinaigrette over the top, top with crumbled feta and finely chopped parsley. Thinly slice half a red onion, and place on the side.

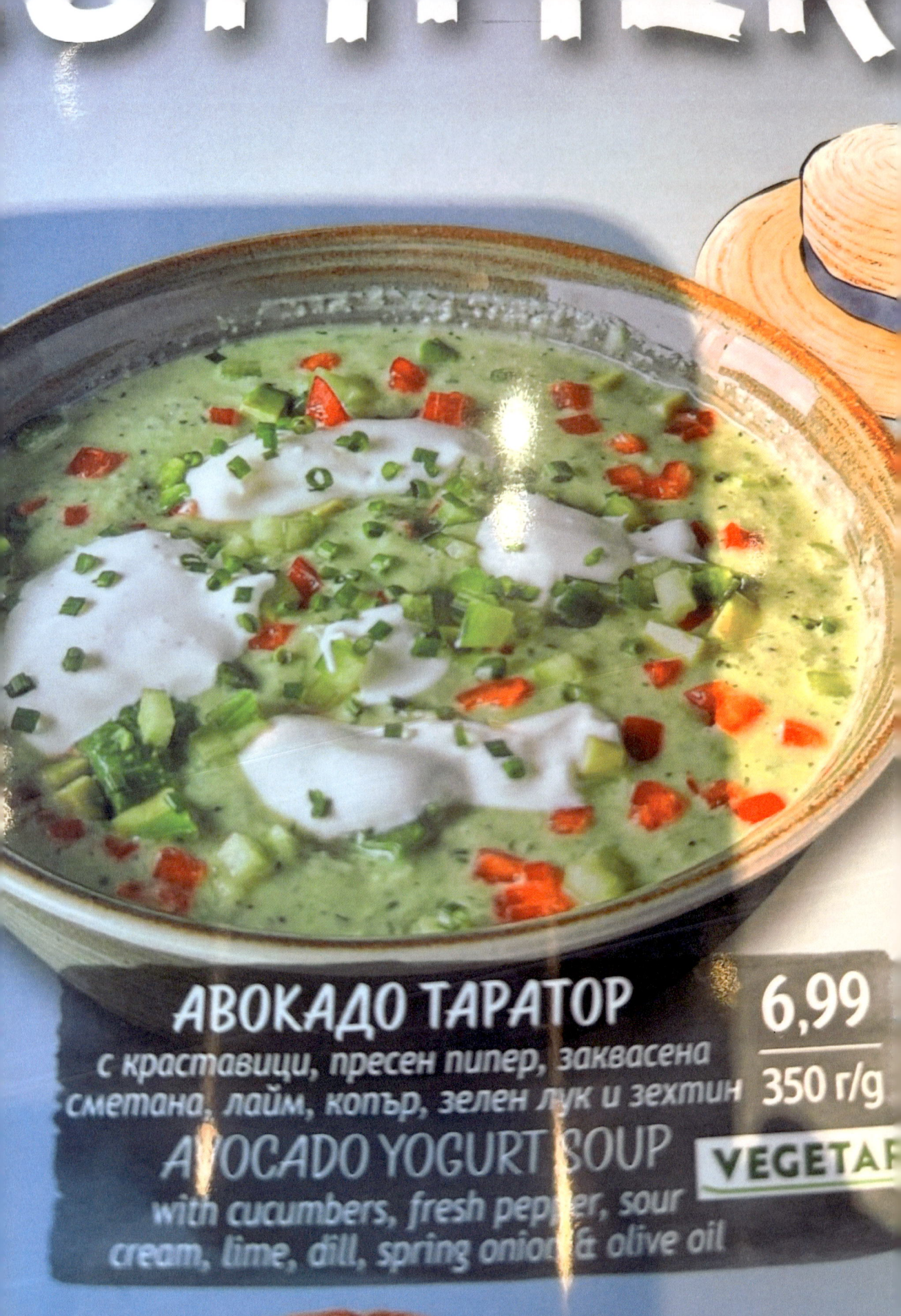

АВОКАДО ТАРАТОР

с краставици, пресен пипер, заквасена
сметана, лайм, копър, зелен лук и зехтин

AVOCADO YOGURT SOUP

with cucumbers, fresh pepper, sour
cream, lime, dill, spring onion & olive oil

6,99

350 г/g

VEGETAR[...]

Avocado Tarator - Cold Summer Soup

INGREDIENTS

One avocado, one cucumber, two cups of Greek or whole milk yogurt, sour cream, half green and red peppers, lime, one spring onion, olive oil, walnuts.

Mash and mix the avocado with the cucumber finely chopped in small squares or grated, the finely chopped ½ green and red peppers in the yogurt. Add a teaspoon of olive oil and walnuts and mix with the yogurt mixture, sprinkle with the finely cut spring onion and dill, sprinkle with lime. Top with two tablespoons of sour cream. Bon appetit!

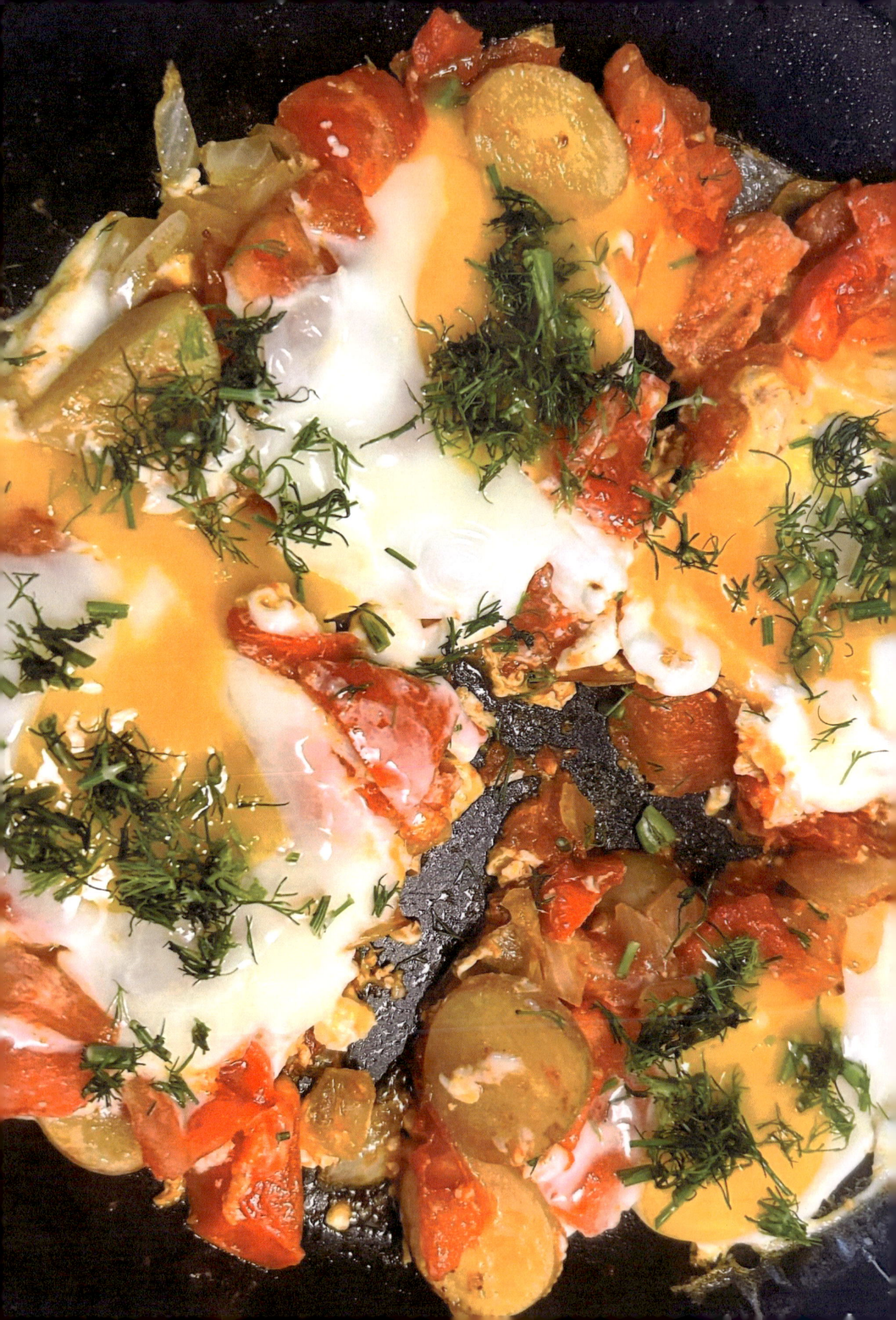

Summer Vegetarian Dish

INGREDIENTS

Two red peppers, two tomatoes, one onion, six small potatoes, four eggs, salt, pepper, savery, dill, olive oil.

Dice the peppers, slice the onions in thin layers and cut the small potatoes in half, cook in a covered pot greased with oil at low heat for 10 min, stir once; dice the tomatoes and add to the pan. Add and mix the spices into the food. Cook at low heat until not watery.

Crack the four eggs on top, each at one of the four sides of the pan, and cook on low heat for another 10 min. Sprinkle with dill.

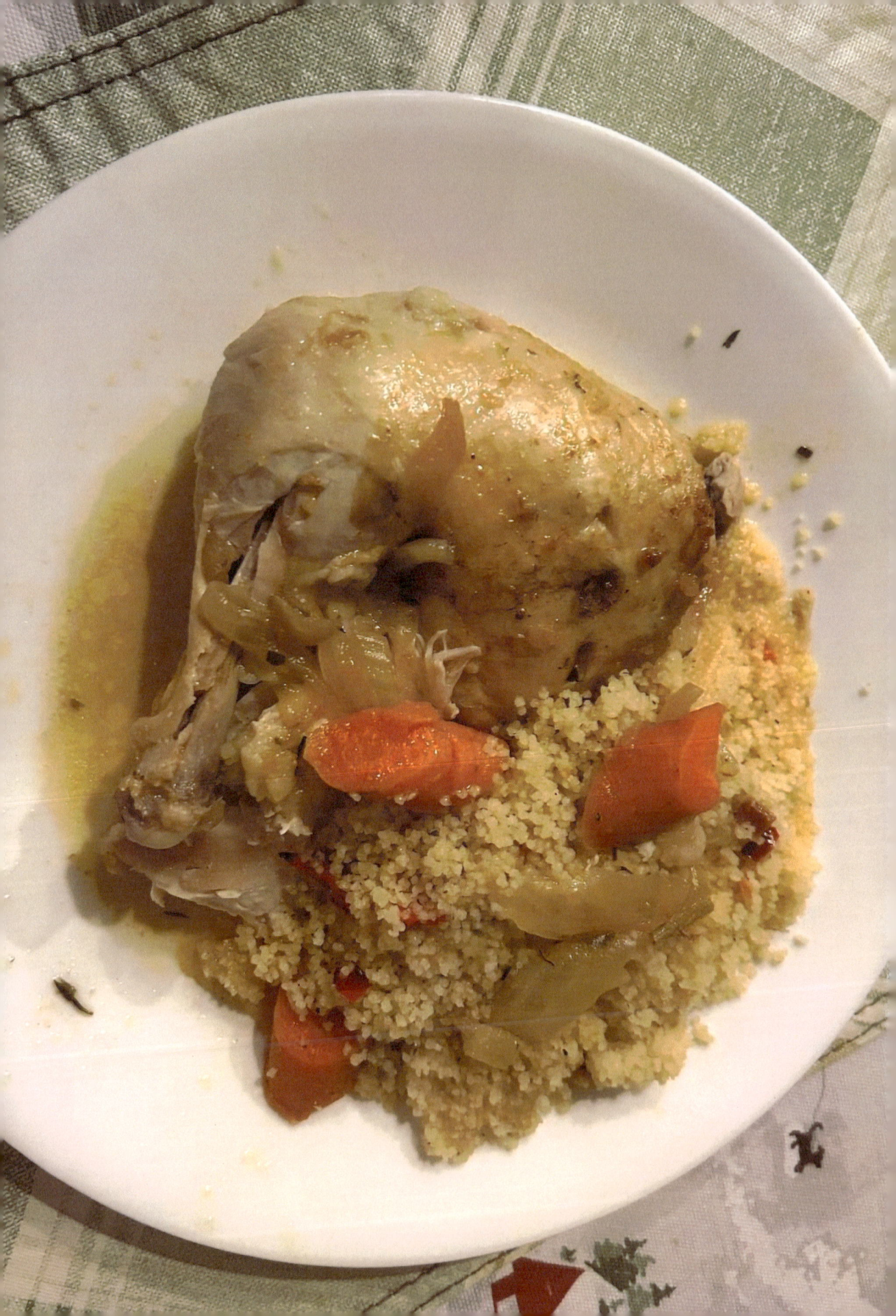

Drunken Chicken with Couscous

INGREDIENTS

One small chicken, a can of beer, a tablespoon of olive oil, two cups of vegetable broth, two carrots, one onion, salt, pepper, sweet paprika, parsley.

Take out the package with chicken livers and heart from the inside of the chicken, wash the chicken well inside and out, and rub with a mixture of oil, salt, pepper and paprika all over it and the cavity. Pour the beer in the cavity of the chicken and place it in a covered baking pan.

Arrange sliced carrots and onion around the chicken. Pour the cups of vegetable broth evenly over the vegetables. Cover and bake at 425 for an hour. Excess chicken broth can be saved for another dish.

Couscous

I usually buy couscous at Sprouts food market in a box with spices inside it. The directions to cook the couscous are to place a cup and ½ of water with the spices and ½ tablespoon of olive oil in a covered dish in the microwave and cook until the water boils (3-4 min). Then stir in the couscous. Cover, wait for 5 min. Fluff with a fork and it's ready to serve.

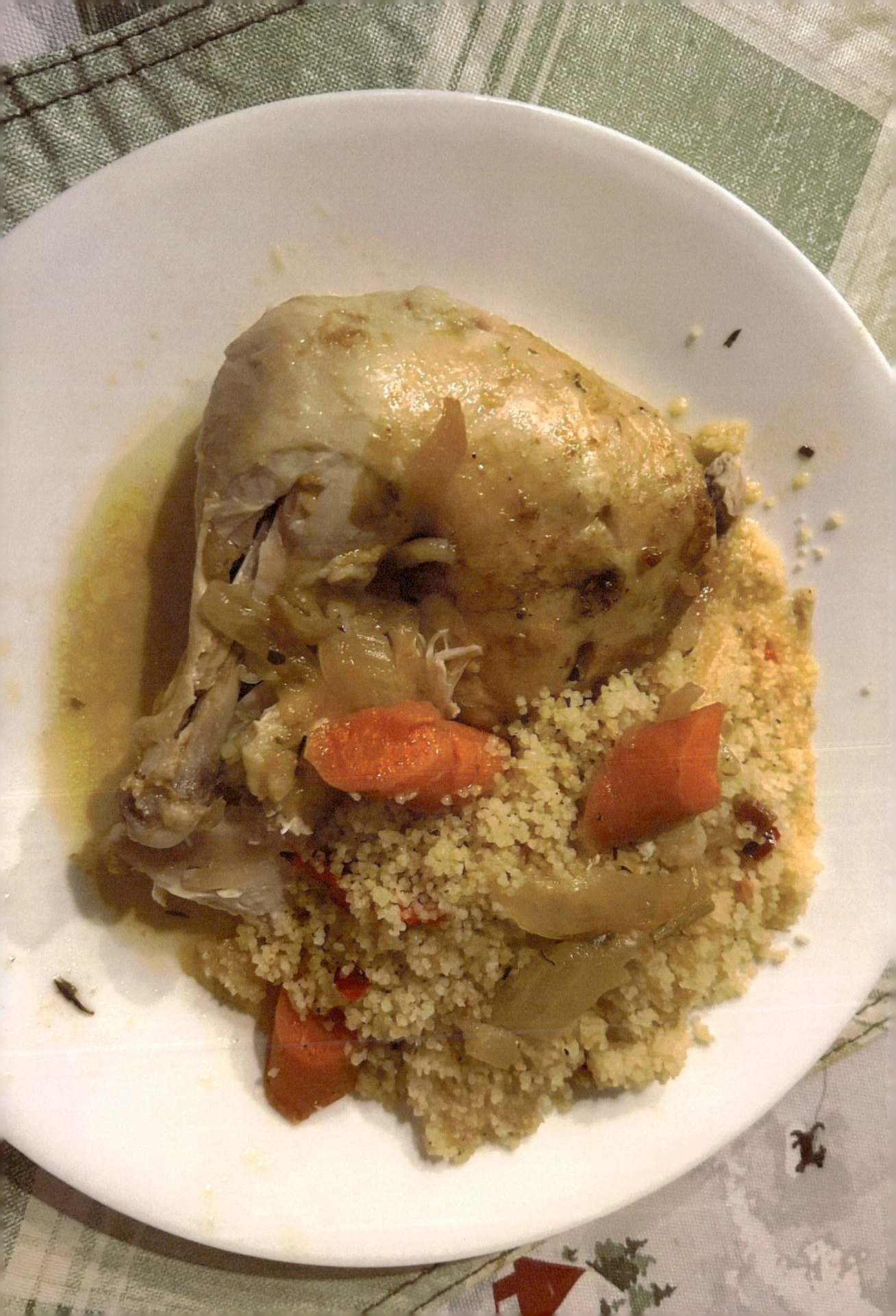

Moroccan couscous

Couscous, a cup and ½ water, olive oil, salt, pepper.

Place water and olive oil in a pot. Bring the water to a boil. Take off the stove, toss in the couscous, cover and let sit for five minutes. Fluff with a fork. Place on the bottom of the serving dish, followed by the chicken and the vegetables, pour the sauce on top.

www.ingramcontent.com/pod-product-compliance
Lightning Source LLC
Chambersburg PA
CBRC090838120626
46551CB00008B/693